THE SELF-SHIATSU HANDBOOK

THE SELF-SHIATSU HANDBOOK

PAMELA FERGUSON

Photography by Alison Russell

A PERIGEE BOOK

A Perigee Book
Published by The Berkley Publishing Group
200 Madison Avenue
New York, NY 10016

Copyright © 1995 by Pamela Ferguson

Back cover and interior photographs by Alison Russell.
Graphic arts by Friedrich Hartmann, Nagold. Copyright © Georg Thieme Verlag, Stuttgart 1995.

Photograph models: Ellen Barfield, Martha Bowers, Nancy Edgar, Larry Egbert, Patty Horii, Michael
Jolly, Monica Jolly, Gregory Jones, Daphne Lewis, Sandra Lugo-Camacho, Gauri Mehta, Shreefal Mehta,
Oralia Ortiz, Kumar Pallana, Isabelle Selassie, William Smith, Bernadette Winiker, Phyllis Wood,
Kathryn Wood, Louis Wood, Bryce Wood.

Book design by H Roberts Design
Cover design by James R. Harris
Front cover photograph by Jill Levine

First edition: August 1995

Published simultaneously in Canada.
The German language edition is simultaneously published by TRIAS – Thieme Hippokrates Enke.
Copyright © Georg Thieme Verlag, Stuttgart 1995.

**This book is not intended as a substitute for the medical advice of physicians. The reader should
regularly consult a physician about matters relating to his or her health and particularly regard-
ing any symptom that may require diagnosis or medical attention.**

Library of Congress Cataloging-in-Publication Data
Ferguson, Pamela.
    The self-shiatsu handbook / Pamela Ferguson.
        p.   cm.
    "A Perigee book."
    Includes bibliographical references and index.
    ISBN 0–399–51949–1
    1. Acupressure.   I.   Title
RM723.A27F47   1995
615.8'22—dc20   94–23816
                                                                          CIP

Printed in the United States of America

10 9 8 7 6 5 4 3 2 1

This book is printed on acid-free paper.
∞

To the teachers and pupils of the Etafeni grassroot educational projects

of Cape Town, who taught me that schools can be created

by a few kindred spirits under an open African sky.

CONTENTS

FOREWORD

Shiatsu changed my life and my medical practice.

I have known Pamela Ferguson for twelve years, as an excellent teacher who came to Montreal to train shiatsu therapists.

Thoroughly imbued with Western thinking and Cartesian doctrine, my analytical left brain found it weird that the bladder could be stimulated through the little toe, or the stomach through the upper leg. But with quiet conviction, Pam patiently explained the autonomic nervous system, the meridian paths, yin and yang. She showed us how migraines occurred, since the associated meridian of the gallbladder is, among other things, on a double parietal and occipital line.

Today, now that I in turn am qualified to teach shiatsu, it is my pleasure to explain the meridians to my patients. They too can use the right pressure points to relieve their varying ailments. Self-shiatsu in the morning sets a vital energy in motion. Sedentary jobs that keep people hunched over a computer screen cause pain in the nape of the neck and shoulders. By regular pressure we can reduce the tension and discomfort and ultimately make them disappear.

When I was expecting a baby, I received a shiatsu treatment every two weeks throughout my pregnancy. The teacher-therapist sensed my child would be a girl because of her high "yin" energy. But I did not want to accept this. According to official Western medicine, the ultrasound picture at seventeen weeks, I was expecting a boy. Imagine my joy to discover a splendid, bright little girl, and one so calm! Sometimes technology needs a helping hand from intuition.

I am sure that shiatsu had a beneficial effect on my unborn child and on her immune system. What is more, my daughter was in a breech position until two weeks before the birth. Her father and I practiced the clockwise abdominal exercise (see p. 110, exercise 4) to get her to turn, which she did the day before the birth. I was accompanied throughout the long labor by a shiatsu therapist. My gynecologist considered a cesarean or medication. Neither was needed. With stimulation to the relevant meridians and pressure points, my perineum muscles flexed and the cervix dilated. The birth was normal.

Now seven, my daughter Ariane asks me to put her to sleep using shiatsu. She also knows which meridians to stimulate to prevent colds and flu at the first sign of symptoms.

Thank you, Pamela Ferguson, for having been magician, teacher, friend, and confidante, and for having taught me an art to add to my traditional medical knowledge.

Lise Ste-Marie, M.D.
Longueuil, Quebec

PREFACE

The Self-Shiatsu Handbook is a practical guide for you, your family, and your friends.

This book has evolved over a decade of workshops spanning Montreal, New York, Dallas, New Orleans, Zurich, Winterthur, Basel, Bern, Berlin, Hamburg, Freiburg, Dresden, and Cape Town. My students come from many different backgrounds, but have taught me that aches and pains speak all languages. Throughout the years, students and friends have asked me to consolidate our classes into simplified self-shiatsu texts for themselves, their loved ones, and, where relevant, their patients. Many express a frustration with leading textbooks that are aimed mainly at long-term shiatsu students but do not show enough self-shiatsu techniques for everyday problems like headaches, congestion, or backache.

Weary of painkillers and side effects, they wanted a simple, healthy, and inexpensive way of tackling and preventing chronic pain. Our discussions also provided a supportive framework for shared insights and experiences. Above all, shiatsu was appreciated for its compassionate touch.

Our workshops provide an open forum for experimentation. We apply the ancient art of shiatsu to aches and pains people have suffered from time immemorial and equally to modern problems like computer-related stress and jet lag.

As an itinerent teacher, I also learn as my students share the folk healing customs of their different cultures and the pain-relieving remedies they have worked out for themselves. Our discussions, I hope, add zest, humor, and love to the evolution of an ancient craft. This handbook reflects our workshops. We've taken shiatsu out of its formal setting on a mat or futon on the floor and into the jet age.

A final word about the photographs. You'll catch only an occasional glimpse of my hands and feet. The friends who generously agreed to model for the book range in age from six to eighty, and come from a lively mix of backgrounds and cultures. They include medical doctors, nurses, a radiology technician, engineers, massage therapists, artists, a yoga teacher, an art historian, businesspeople, peace activists, and students.

Most of them had not even heard of shiatsu—let alone practiced it—until I trained them in front of the camera. This was intentional on my part, to show you that anyone can do the techniques they were demonstrating.

Although self-shiatsu and the mini-sessions in this book can never be as comprehensive as a full-body one-hour session from a professionally trained shiatsu therapist, there is ample room, as our models agreed, to revive a simplified form of shiatsu as a folk remedy.

We're offering something totally different here from formal shiatsu school textbook photos of teachers working on students or models. I wanted a change of pace from the "master/pupil" image.

So I hope this will encourage you to see yourself in our photos. Always remember, folk shiatsu mirrors the art that is lying dormant within you. Or, as the Zen saying goes, *Zen is like looking for the spectacles that are sitting on your nose*.

ACKNOWLEDGMENTS

My journey through the art of healing has been inspired by many people: by my meditation teacher, the late Hilda Charlton of New York; by my Zen Shiatsu teachers Pauline Sasaki, Ohashi, and Esther Turnbull; by Tet Saito, president of the Shiatsu Center of Toronto; and by New York chiropractors Linda Li and Dick Kowal. In Montreal, my thanks go to Jean Lecomte, Raymond Ricard, M.D., Suzanne Ricard, R.N., psychologist Claudette LeBlanc, Elisabeth Reichel, M.D., and Lise Ste-Marie, M.D., for building so many bridges between western medicine and shiatsu. My colleagues and friends in Europe, Matthias Wieck, Wilfried Rappenecker, M.D., Erika Bringold, Elli Mann-Langhof, Edith Storch, and Bernhard Ruhla, have dedicated themselves to the growth and spread of shiatsu as a professional discipline requiring years of study. My gratitude goes to Bernadette Winiker, R.N., who planned workshops for me in a number of Swiss hospitals and who provides me with a solid balance between western medicine and my life. To my Swiss physicians Idillio Noseda, M.D., of New York and Verena Hablützel, M.D., of Zurich for their support. To photographer Alison Russell for the wholehearted way she tackled this project during weekends. To those friends who modeled for us and gave so generously of their time. To two great editors, Susanne Warmuth in Stuttgart and Irene Prokop in New York. To my terrific agents Edy Selman in New York and Ruth Weibel in Zurich. Finally, to my students and patients, who will always be my best teachers.

THE SELF-SHIATSU HANDBOOK

Introduction: What Is Shiatsu?

A decade or so ago, people used to say "Shzzz . . . Isn't that some kind of a dog?" when I spoke about shiatsu. Now they nod and say, "Ah, shiatsu. That's something like acupuncture without needles, isn't it?"

In Japanese, *shiatsu* combines two words: *shi* (finger) and *atsu* (pressure): literally, finger pressure. But the name is short for a variety of techniques, rooted in some of the earliest forms of family healing in China which date back thousands of years and involve pressure point work and stretching, which are believed to have been introduced to Japan with the spread of Buddhism. Today there are many different forms of acupressure and shiatsu (Chinese, Korean, and Japanese) and many different schools.

I was trained in a highly structured form of Zen Shiatsu, modernized and updated in this century. Apart from learning different meridians (lines of energy) and dozens of pressure points and stretches, we studied precise ways of selecting combinations of meridians and pressure points according to the need of the receiver. We work with the principles of the five elements. We learn how to center and focus. Like any Zen art or discipline, shiatsu becomes a route, a long route, to enlightenment.

Zen Shiatsu continues to evolve through great teachers like Pauline Sasaki of the United States and her innovative Quantum Shiatsu, and Tetsuro Saito of Canada, whose background in engineering and shiatsu contributed to his discovery of meridian systems that challenge ancient Chinese and twentieth-century Japanese systems.

In Zen Shiatsu we work mainly on our knees on a mat on the floor in traditional postures that are often quite new to those of us raised in Western cultures. Meditation and exercises are at the heart of our training and practice. Many people ask me how long it takes to learn Zen Shiatsu. The answer is years. Basic certification after a couple of years is just the beginning.

Exposure to Zen and its many expressions, through Zazen, calligraphy, the tea ceremony, Japanese teahouse architecture, meditation gardens, martial arts, and so on, offers enriching experiences to a serious student.

But you don't need to journey that long route to understand the simplified, mini-techniques in *The Self-Shiatsu Handbook*.

Apart from teaching curricula at different schools of shiatsu and Chinese medicine, I have sought any and every opportunity to share the art, to demystify and "package" techniques for different workshops, in hospitals, at patients' bedsides, in offices, gyms, women's centers, retirement homes, and for HIV-positive groups.

One impromptu workshop grew out of an English class for literacy teachers near Cape Town.

I taught in East Berlin before the wall fell and happened to be teaching in West Berlin on November 9, 1989, when the wall was opened. I cherish the political discussions that are an ongoing part of our shiatsu classes. Shiatsu is seen as a practical aid, an anchor in times of change and insecurity, and not as some esoteric art practiced only by sages on remote mountaintops in the East.

As the majority of shiatsu students in the West are women, there are many complaints about the condescending tone of certain textbooks and attitudes (found in both Western and Eastern medicine) and the glib way in which so-called women's problems are treated. Our discussions are reflected in the section entitled "Women's Corner."

It has been encouraging, with each year, to see an increasing number of men learning shiatsu, especially in Germany. In my classes we touch some subtle chords in our discussions about the "male cycle," a recognition of the monthly changes or ebb and flow men experience in their own bodies and emotions, a seeming taboo that doesn't appear in medical literature. In my classes men have talked intimately and poetically about such cyclic changes. For some, this was the first sharing in a mixed setting of feelings they felt as boys, which their parents recognized only in their sisters.

The blunting effect of a macho upbringing hits many levels. I don't see men networking and campaigning for more awareness and research funds for prostate and testicular cancer in the way women campaign for breast cancer. Men constitute about 1 percent of breast cancer cases, but that end of the subject, sadly, is a whispered taboo.

Our workshops help to air taboos.

Along with all aspects of sexism, we also discuss the effects of pollution, poverty, and racism on community health. We open windows on menopause, breast cancer, and AIDS. We discuss the role shiatsu can play to raise a sense of consciousness, and compassion, heal divisions, and offer an inner calm in the midst of a troubled world.

PRACTICAL SHIATSU

In its complete form, shiatsu looks like a graceful harmonization of acupressure and stretching, involving a similar pressure point and meridian system to acupuncture. No needles, oils, or creams are used, as the receiver is fully clothed. Techniques can be slow and subtle, or brisk, involving thumb, palm, or elbow pressure.

Shiatsu is not massage. The philosophy is different, and so is the touch.

Let's glimpse back in time to the origin of shiatsu as a folk remedy.

You all practice an instinctive form of self-shiatsu each time you press your forehead to relieve a headache, or pinch the bridge of your nose to ease eyestrain, or rub your arms briskly when you feel cold. You not only stimulate relevant lines of energy (meridians) and pressure points, but you are accessing some of the earliest and most ancient forms of healing and preventive care.

The pressure you use in those instinctive exercises should be a guide to you when you practice some of the techniques in this book. There's a subtle art in applying pressure slowly and evenly to avoid pain and resistance. Practice on yourself first before you practice on others. Press down slowly, hold to a count of five, and release slowly. Don't make the common mistake of thinking you have to wiggle your thumb or make rapid circular movements to be effective. You don't. You just press in and hold. You stop time.

Some of you will prefer a light pressure. Others can take quite a deep pressure. You will soon find out what works best for you. Shiatsu is a peaceful and concentrated technique, as you will discover the more you practice it.

Try this simple exercise. Inhale and exhale slowly. Raise your hands, palms facing one another. Gradually move them together and apart, without touching.

Move in slow motion. Keep your eyes closed if this helps you concentrate. In time you may feel a magnetic pull between your palms. Keep going. That magnetic force will grow the more you do this exercise. Now find a tense or tight muscle on your leg. Place your hands on it and feel the warmth. Then place your thumb on it and press down gradually. Don't jab. Don't be in a hurry. The slower you press, the deeper you can go. Hold the point, count to five. Release slowly. Repeat the exercise a couple of times. Now move an inch or so along the tight muscle, and try again. Move on another inch, and try again.

With practice, you may feel increasing warmth, tingling, a release of tension or pain.

In shiatsu this is explained in terms of stimulating or releasing blocked ki (*qi* or *chi* in Chinese), translated as energy or life force. In the West we have to be taught ki. In the East ki is part of the lingo, meaning breath, energy, spirit, the vitality or intelligence that propels the universe and makes us tick.

In Japanese the transliteration *Genki desuka*, "How are you?" is "How is your ki?" Even weather conditions are described as variations in ki.

Students steeped in Western medicine try to relate ki to the nervous system, by saying acupuncture and shiatsu hit nerve centers to block pain perception. Others equate ki with ATP (adenosine triphosphate), the powerhouse of the cell, the essential molecule that is the energy currency of living systems. Some describe the stimulation of ki as a stimulation of endorphins, the body's own painkillers, to explain the feeling of calm and well-being after shiatsu. One of the best scientific records of ki involves Kirlian photography, showing an increase of magnetic energy patterns around pressure points after shiatsu or acupuncture.

But ki transcends all these explanations. We don't have a simple translation for it in the West. In yoga we refer to ki as *prana*, and a similar understanding of a universal life force is awakened in us when we meditate or do breathing exercises. Working with ki involves focus, an insight into the essence of oriental healing as a process of balancing opposites and discords in the body and in the universe. So, too, the arts of tai chi, qi gong, and aikido involve raising and harmonizing ki.

Faced with skeptics in my classes, I throw theory to the wind. I ask people to pair up and start working on tight shoulders. Experience, I remind them, predates theoretical explanations.

Let your body be your teacher. You don't have to believe in ki for shiatsu to work.

Our instinctive understanding of the body as a communication or electromagnetic system is conveyed through expressions like "My batteries have run down" or "This turns me on/turns me off" or "I feel burned out" or "I'm suffering from overload." All matter is energy in motion, and our bodies vibrate at different frequencies of ki, according to Eastern medical philosophy. To put it more simply, ki is organized along vertical pathways or meridians in a grid that resembles a subway or bus system.

Meridians relate to physiology, emotions, and the psyche.

Pressure points lining those meridians resemble bus stops, stations, or junctions.

We all know what it's like when routes become congested or trains break down. We all curse traffic jams or delays at stations or airports. If we're lucky, other systems absorb the overload, people are rerouted, but further congestions can occur, especially at peak hour. Similar things happen in the human body. Our circuits, our meridians, become backed up, overloaded in some areas and emptied in other areas. The use of acupuncture needles or thumb pressure helps to unclog congestion or jump-start stagnant energy. To put it another way, if a light goes off in your room, the problem could be local (a bulb), or perhaps you've blown a fuse or your wiring is faulty.

Thus we may ease a headache by pressing the forehead, the sacrum, or the big toe.

Advanced texts on Eastern medicine use more esoteric explanations, of course, all of which will become more understandable if you choose to go beyond the scope of this book.

You'll notice I have avoided naming the pressure points and meridians (lines) according to acupuncture and shiatsu systems, because at this stage it's more important for you to discover them through touch and get to know them as good buddies. Often, your thumb will slide right into the points. Some will feel snug and comforting. Some will be more sensitive than others. Some will feel tight and painful. Adjust your pressure accordingly.

The more you work with them, the more they will reveal to you. Sometimes, just holding one pressure point, with concentration, can change the flow of energy in your entire body and teach you as much about your body as a grain of sand or a snow crystal can teach you about the universe.

Students often ask, Do meridians flow along or between the muscles? Along veins or arteries? Do they correspond to the lymphatic system? Or the autonomic nervous system? Or the organs perhaps? Meridians relate to all of these and more in function, but not in location, with some exceptions.

To appreciate meridians, try to backtrack several thousand years in your mind to a time that predates our formal Western knowledge of anatomy and physiology, when the body was viewed as a microcosm of the universe, the elements and seasons, and studied in terms of the ebb and flow of energies. People listened to their bodies and stretched a limb or two to wake up or to ease pain. They pressed points that hurt, only to discover that the points had many other functions besides easing a local pain. They discovered that a headache could be eased by pressing points on the feet, or menstrual pain could be eased by pressing points below the knee and above the ankle. The longer I teach, the more convinced I become of a universality of simple pressure point work (often combined with herbology) passed down from generation to generation in the oldest cultures of East and West.

After teaching certain exercises in my classes, how often have I heard a voice say, "My grandmother used to do that to us as kids." The voices were Korean, Irish, Vietnamese, Indian, Palestinian, Iranian, Native American, Caribbean, and African.

PART I

UNDERSTANDING PAIN

We all have niggling aches and pains.

Some 90 million Americans suffer from chronic pain, according to the National Institutes of Health in Washington.

Some become addicted to painkillers. Others spend an estimated $13 billion annually in seeking relief through alternative treatments: chiropractic, acupuncture, aroma therapy, biofeedback, homeopathy, reflexology, shiatsu, or different combinations of these. But many people don't tell their family doctors, for fear of ridicule or anger. A lack of "scientific proof" is often given as the main argument against alternatives, with no distinction made between methods like acupuncture, that are thousands of years old, and some new gimmick with a fancy name.

But things are evolving as the field of preventive medicine broadens with changes in the health system. A tiny but growing number of physicians integrate alternatives with conventional treatment, the best of both worlds, in a quest for a more holistic approach. Shiatsu or acupuncture methods are often sought as a last resort for patients who cannot receive further painkillers or who don't respond to them.

Harvard Medical School was the first of about six medical schools in the United States to offer courses in alternatives. Harvard professors of behavioral medicine have long-established links with traditional Chinese medicine, well documented by Harvard's David Eisenberg, M.D., in his book *Encounters with Qi*, following his own internship in acupuncture clinics in China.

During 1993 Bill Moyers' popular *Healing and the Mind* series on American public television (PBS) described the effectiveness of meditation to ease pain and stress at a stress clinic at the University of Massachusetts Medical Center, Boston, and the value of support groups for chronic pain, cancer survivors, and the terminally ill. Yale surgeon and author Dr. Bernie S. Siegel revolutionized cancer treatment with patient involvement and positive imagery.

Pain experts like Dr. Darrell Tanelian, director of the pain management center at the University of Texas Southwestern Medical Center, Dallas, also talk about the need to wean patients off the "quick shot" or "instant pill" solution. A keen rollerblader and fitness addict, he emphasizes patient input involving change of diet, exercise, and lifestyle to combat pain.

Even more encouraging, the National Institutes of Health recently created an office of alternative medicine to document information and fund research.

Current NIH research projects at medical schools and centers nationwide include tai chi (for balance disorders), qi gong (for dystrophy), yoga (for obsessive-compulsive disorders), imagery (to boost immune system), hypnosis (for low-back pain), and acupuncture (for unipolar depression and hyperactivity).

Hopefully, the results of these studies will speed up the integration of alternatives with mainstream medicine, more in line with some European countries. Most pharmacies in Germany and Switzerland offer *Kräuterheilkunde*—a knowledge of herbal healing. Natural remedies or herbal concoctions can be bought over the counter, and insurance pays if a physician prescribes them. People who practice shiatsu, acupuncture, or herbology often become formally licensed as a *Heilpraktiker/in* (natural healer). My classes have included surgeons (heart and orthopedic) and family physicians who also practice reflexology, music therapy, and ear acupuncture. Complementary medicine as it is known in Britain has a long tradition, and acupuncture was first used there in the seventeenth century. Some of London's teaching hospitals offer alternatives (including shiatsu) under the national health service in outpatient clinics, not only for pain control but for HIV patients and for recovering addicts. Inner-city funding has helped finance the Hoxton Health Group, offering shiatsu, acupuncture, and homeopathy to senior citizens three days a week for a nominal monthly fee at St. Leonards Hospital in Hackney.

Alternative practitioners even offer their services on a pay-what-you-can basis one night each week in the crypt under St. James's Church, Piccadilly, in the heart of London. Which means hundreds have access to treatments they may not otherwise be able to afford.

During years of teaching in Montreal, Canada, I noticed the growth of *médecine douce* ("soft" medicine). As part of the outreach internship program at Shiatsu-Ki Quebec school, we were able to arrange for advanced students to work on patients in local hospitals, especially on men and women who were chronically disabled and bedridden and had no families.

Over the years, my students in Canada, Germany, and Switzerland have included an increasing number of physicians, nurses, midwives, psychologists, and especially physiotherapists, in regular classes and in special workshops.

Many come, not just to acquire a new technique, but to seek stress and pain release for themselves. We learn from one another. We learn about pain from different perspectives. At no time is shiatsu presented as a panacea or some magic cure, but as a method to integrate and try, especially when a patient cannot receive more pain medication. Shiatsu is also a great tool for health professionals who believe in the importance of a gentle, healing touch to balance high-tech or invasive procedures.

And this underlines the vital essence of shiatsu. It gives joy. It feels good. I emphasize this when teaching physiotherapists, in particular: that they start their sessions with a few shiatsu techniques and breathing exercises to help release and relax patients and give them a sense of joy and uplift. I suggest they work on the healthy side of the body first—or the feet—before tackling the injured or restricted limb or problem area.

Subsequent procedures move more smoothly. The patient is more relaxed and less resistant. Pain is minimized. Above all, joy and laughter are great healers and immune system boosters, as we learned from Norman Cousins' classic work *Anatomy of an Illness*.

It's been fascinating to see how the integration of shiatsu and other alternatives changes health professionals. M.D.'s choose softer colors and soothing artwork for their offices and clinics. They use more books and visual aids to discuss medical details with patients. They stop wearing white, swap black stethoscopes for red, purchase instruments in softer materials, place floral fabrics over the metal stirrups on their gynecological exam tables.

Nurses squeeze a few moments into their busy schedules to help pain, insomnia, and constipation by applying just a few shiatsu techniques on patients, instead of relying on pain medications. Midwives, in particular, have been able to make great use of shiatsu techniques during home births.

But a medical background is not a prerequisite for learning shiatsu. My students range from dancers to schoolteachers, bakers to ceramicists, politicians to construction workers, housewives to househusbands, to the unemployed. Some are seeking a shift in their lives, some are seeking second careers, and others just want techniques they can utilize with their families. They often ask if a particular belief system is required for shiatsu to be effective.

The answer is no, absolutely not.

I tell them how my own life led me to shiatsu via a circuitous route. At the age of six in Cornwall, I was told by a Gypsy palmist that I had healing hands. Other fortune-tellers in different parts of the world said the same thing throughout the years, but I took it all with a grain of salt. I still do. In shiatsu we view the hands as vehicles for ki, and not as a source.

I also remember (though it meant little at the time) an amazing day with my great-aunt Ena at her 300-year-old cottage built on several levels of a slope in the coastal village of Marazion in Cornwall. We stood in her walled garden overlooking the sea and a view of the legendary isle of St. Michael's Mount, where hermits once dwelled, and where ancient Phoenicians used to trade in tin.

She pointed at her fruit trees, vegetables, and herb garden, fragrant with mint, chamomile, sage, thyme, and rosemary, and a lawn dotted with daisies and dandelion. "Everything I need to heal me is either in this garden or in my body," she said, as gulls wheeled overhead in the salty breeze.

"I can see what's in the garden, but what's planted in your body?" I asked.

"Don't be facetious, young lady. The body is its own pharmacy. If we know which buttons to tap."

Great-Aunt Ena was a gifted storyteller, so I put all this down to Cornish folklore. Until a few years later.

During the 1970s when I was an ambitious journalist and writer, I had two interesting experiences that prove we all have a shiatsu-like blueprint buried deep in our collective unconscious. A friend of mine, an eye surgeon in London, suffered from chronic back pain, and nothing seemed to help. One day I made a V-for-victory sign with my first and second fingers, pressed two points on either side of his spine, and the pain vanished.

A couple of years later in San Francisco, and after a shift into meditation, yoga, and vegetarianism as a way of balancing a stressful career, I happened to numb Sophie Keir's toothache by reaching out and holding a point on her arm. It didn't solve the problem, of course, but it did enable her to travel by bus, pain-free, to see the dentist. Later she happened to come across Shizuto Masunaga's classic *Zen Shiatsu* in a Japanese bookshop.

"You want to know what happened to my toothache? Read this," she said, tossing me the book. We had never even heard of shiatsu before. But interestingly enough, we were living opposite an acupuncture center. And I was deeply impressed by the calming effect of people performing tai chi in a nearby park where I jogged each morning.

The city was trying to teach me something. Within a year I started my training at the Shiatsu Education Center (now the Ohashi Institute) in New York City and my entire life changed.

I was writing my fifth book at the time and thought shiatsu would be a useful hobby. But it evolved into a second career. After graduating, I joined the teaching staff for a couple of years before branching out on my own.

For the last decade I've been fortunate enough to see shiatsu grow in the West, especially through the pioneering work of Tet Saito, Pauline Sasaki, and Ohashi, and the enterprising shiatsu schools developed by Jean Lecomte of Montreal; Erika Bringold of Winterthur, Switzerland; Matthias Wieck, Elli Mann-Langhof, and Edith Storch of Berlin; Wilfried Rappenecker of Hamburg; and Bernhard Ruhla of Dresden. I have grown through their growth and vision. Some came to shiatsu via medical careers; others came via careers ranging from architecture to chemistry to language teaching to graphic art.

My background as an investigative journalist in a number of different countries and political situations gave me a rare insight into humanity, pain, stress, and survival, invaluable training for the art of healing. Journalism teaches one how to ask questions, and to read silences, an art that is often sadly lacking in medical training. I have also experienced many of the pains we discuss in this book. I encourage my students to utilize their own aches and pains and personal experiences with illness as a training ground, a home laboratory, rich with insights and solutions. Edward E. Rosenbaum, M.D., chronicled his own remarkable evolution through cancer in *The Doctor*.

As I wrote most of my books on battered old portables hauled around the world in pre-laptop days, I know what it's like to work hours at a desk and suffer from chronic back pain. I now know what it's like to suffer from eyestrain, disorientation, and neck tension after hours at a computer keyboard, prompting me to develop exercises to prevent such problems. Jogging taught me a lot about the origin of key pressure points in the legs. Yoga taught me the importance of certain points to keep the knees supple. Migraines run in my family, so I've been able to help several migraine sufferers based on the techniques that help me.

Because I've spent my life crisscrossing the Atlantic, traveling has prompted me to experiment with a series of exercises to overcome jet lag.

I also happen to be a breast cancer survivor. No, shiatsu does not cure cancer, but shiatsu's related disciplines in meditation, focus, and energy-field exercises have been part of my survival kit.

I am living proof of the value of integrating mainstream with alternative medicine, in healing cancer that had metastasized. I had surgery, followed by five years of mistletoe (Iscador) immunotherapy, and a year of modified chemotherapy. Prophetically, I wrote a book about the tobacco industry and lung cancer after reporting on the industry in London years before my own cancer was diagnosed. Prophetically, too, I gave shiatsu to breast cancer survivors long before my mastectomy. Which meant I had the groundwork to become better informed.

So this book mixes shiatsu theory with the raw life experiences I have since been able to transform into teaching material.

Self-shiatsu is most effective when it prompts a process of learning and discovery of the mosaic of factors that trigger chronic aches and pains. The key here is involvement and control. Self-shiatsu works best at the first glimmer of pain, or as prevention. As with any home remedy, use it with discretion and common sense and not as some push-button cure-all.

Seek a physician's advice if in any doubt.

A . STRESS

Stress is our worst enemy. We all suffer from stress-related aches and pains. Understanding stress is halfway to understanding its spin-offs: chronic pain and illness.

But there are no instant solutions. Not everyone has access to yoga or meditation classes, health clubs, clean swimming pools, cycling paths, golf, or relaxing hobbies, although all help offset twentieth-century stress. Faced with the daily realities of a nasty boss, unemployment, debts, toxic waste, a sick child or parent, a difficult relationship, or high-pressure work, we can try to develop our own survival skills and outlets by creating peaceful moments as buffers during the day.

A few basic exercises can help clear the channels, release some strain, improve coping mechanisms, and help us find solutions. Crushed in a New York bus or subway at peak hour, I find that a few meditative moments work miracles and create inner space and a pacifying effect on people encircling me.

When confronting a difficult situation or individual, I try to hold love in my heart, not to be holier than thou, but because love provides amazing inner strength, detachment, and solutions. I try to utilize anger as a powerful energy to fuel creativity and activism.

Don't be fooled by false mystics who tell you that anger isn't "spiritual." We've seen too much damage done to health by anger, stress, or sadness turned inward when people are programmed into silence or submission.

Give some of the following exercises a try during a stressful day. See which work best for you.

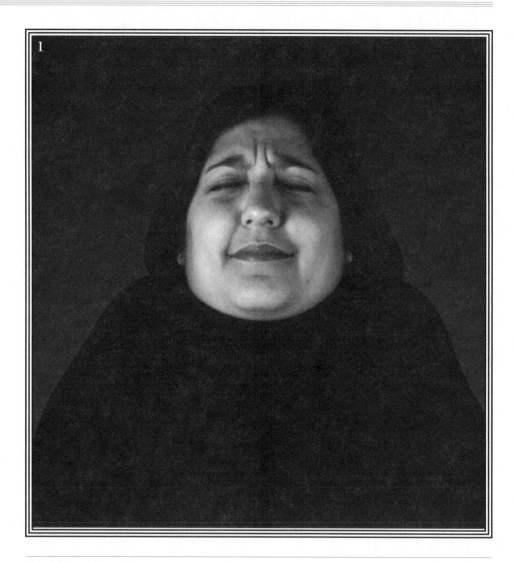

Anti-Stress Exercises

1. Hunch and drop your shoulders a couple of times, then rotate them to ease that "tortoise" syndrome of hunched shoulders and a compressed neck.
2. Sit for a moment, close your eyes, and breathe deeply.
3. Look up and stretch your arms, reaching for the sky, first with one hand, then the other.

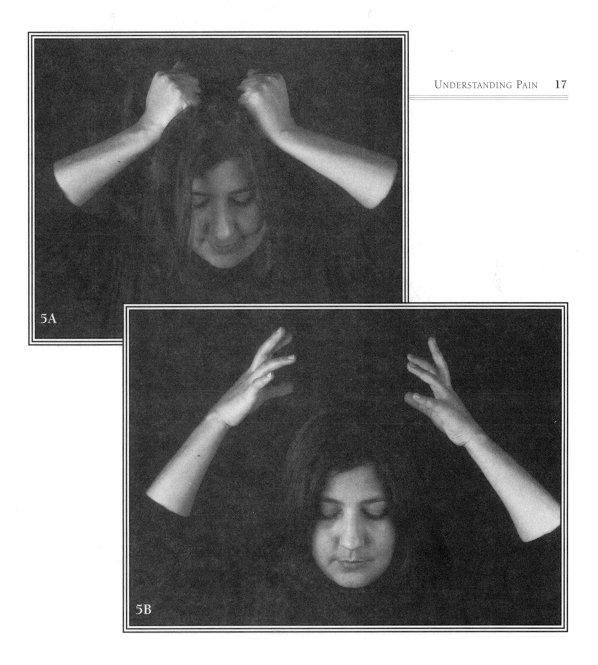

4. Rub your head briskly. Tap it all over with your fingertips.

5A. Tug your hair.

5B. Then release your hands, poof!

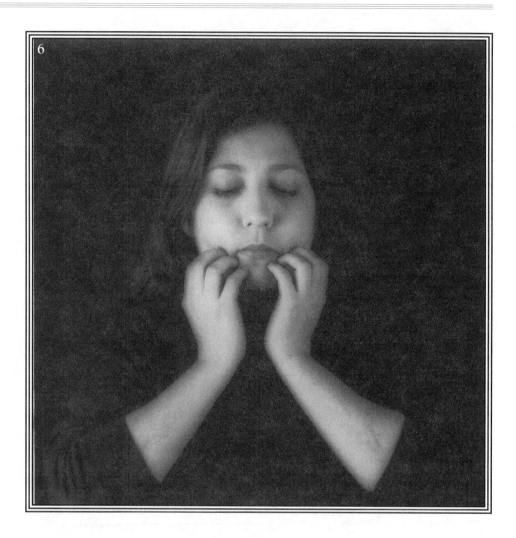

6. Squeeze around your jawline. Tap your jawline. (Both these exercises are good for jaw clenchers and teeth grinders.)
7. Clench your jaw. Open your mouth wide. Imagine you are on the stage of the Metropolitan Opera House or La Scala and say AAAAAH!
8. Squeeze your eyes shut and open them wide. Repeat.
9. Close your eyes while you inhale and exhale slowly, concentrating on the flow of air through your nostrils. If you can, picture something peaceful and beautiful, a flower, a line of poetry, the face of a loved one.

In time, and with practice, such exercises can become a daily habit, something to do (in your mind if necessary) when you're at a bus stop or waiting in line at the post office or supermarket.

As an antistress tool, creative visualization can be practical and fun. If you're caught in traffic and late for an appointment, don't panic. Visualize all the traffic lights turning green. If you're circling the streets hunting for a parking space, visualize one opening up for you. If you're late for a train, struggling along the platforms weighed down by luggage, stop the clock in your mind, freeze it at five minutes before departure time. I swear by this.

Visualization works best when you're focused and don't allow your "monkey mind" to jump around and confuse you.

Once you have tried out all the above suggestions, you'll soon discover which work best for your own personal survival kit.

B. HEADACHES

Headaches are perhaps the most common form of pain, ranging all the way from the mildly distracting to rip-roaring migraines. Migraines run in my family, so I've experienced the worst, not just splitting headaches, but nausea, disorientation, and distorted vision that turns the world into jagged lines or a Francis Bacon painting of concave one-eyed figures.

As with any form of chronic pain, it's useful to keep a pain journal or jot down occurrences on a wall calendar. Note the time, date, place, event, and the food you ate that day.

Note other factors, too, like family arguments or visits from your in-laws. Over a couple of months you may be able to recognize recurring patterns to help you pinpoint or understand triggering factors. Headaches of all forms can be triggered by consuming red wine, chocolate, heavy cream, coffee, cheese, fried bacon, or rich foods.

Women who experience migraines a few days before menstruation have found relief by avoiding meat and dairy products, drinking vegetable juices, and exercising frequently.

Migraines can also be triggered by sensory overload, or by a flickering candle, too much TV or computer work, a photo flash, throbbing disco lights, eye-teasing zigzag or polka-dot patterns, or tropical sunlight bouncing off a white wall.

I can recall experiencing one of my worst migraines in the midst of all the buzzing neon signs and crowds in Berlin's Europa Center on the Kurfürstendamm.

Certain winds or shifts in air pressure can trigger headaches and migraines as well. In Zürich, Switzerland, my head tells me when the dry wind (the Föhn) approaches from the south. Thun (near Bern) is known as headache city, as it catches the brunt of the Föhn. In Cape Town, South Africa, one of the world's windiest cities, my head tells me when the blustery southeaster is on its way.

Self-shiatsu helps to short-circuit pain at the first warning signals or the instant tension starts to creep up the back of the neck. If I don't catch mine early enough, I find it useful to drink a strong cup of tea or put my head under a hot shower. Among my migraine-suffering friends, Uta Brandl of Berlin swears by freshly squeezed orange juice and cold showers; Willy Naidoo of Cape Town swears by tea made of freshly picked peppermint leaves and honey, or indigenous, vitamin-C-and-mineral-rich rooibos tea (sold as Masai tea in Germany). Zuhdi Tarazi, who comes from an old Palestinian Jerusalem family, remembers his mother and grandmother holding nails against points on their foreheads to ease headaches.

While researching headache patterns in Texas and Mexico for a Ph.D. thesis, Isabela Sardas, a young Brazilian psychologist, met village women in Mexico who sip orange tea and place ice cubes or a poultice of clay on their heads to relieve pain.

An estimated 45 million people in the United States suffer from migraines. According to *Life* magazine (February 1994), 157 million workdays are lost to headaches each year. Americans spend over $2 billion on over-the-counter painkillers, and, sadly, the research emphasis is not on prevention, but on finding fancier, more expensive medications.

Awareness of triggering factors is your best way of preventing headaches. I worked with a writer some years ago who suffered daily from headaches. His physician told him there was nothing seriously wrong and suggested he seek relief through an alternative method to wean himself off painkillers.

I taught him every technique in the headache repertory, but nothing seemed to help. I drew on all my own experiences as a writer accustomed to desk- and computer-related stress to suggest pre- and postwork exercises. That didn't work. I suggested he keep a headache journal, so he could note the time of day and any recurring pattern related to food or drink. A few weeks later he called and said he'd discovered the source of his problem.

Chocolate.

He quit his usual chocolate bar a day and his headaches vanished.

Later I repeated this story during one of my classes in Switzerland, haven of Lindt Sprüngli, Suchard, and Toblerone.

Stony silence.

"*Ja, aber,*" came a skeptical voice from the back of the class, "he must have been eating American chocolate."

ANTI-HEADACHE EXERCISES

Shiatsu works best as a preventive measure for headaches. Daily self-shiatsu techniques, coupled with some neck rolls and stretches, especially side stretches, will help relax your neck and shoulders and clear the circuits. Be conscious of what happens to your body when you're angry. Be conscious of your posture. Tension headaches are often triggered by the "tortoise" syndrome, hunched shoulders and a compressed neck, all too typical problems of people who work at desks or drawing boards.

Try the techniques the instant you feel a headache (migraine, cluster, or any other kind) is on its way. Press the points to a count of five, release slowly, press again, release. Repeat a few times. Don't jab, don't press too hard. The slower you press, the deeper you can go. If you experience pain on one side, work on the opposite side first.

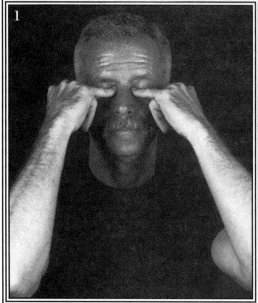

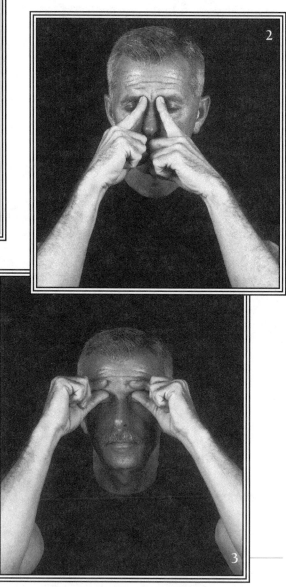

Anti-Headache Exercises

1. Press the inside corners of each eye. Pinch the bridge of your nose.
2. Press points under your eyebrows. Rest your head on your fingertips if necessary.
3. Pinch your eyebrows.

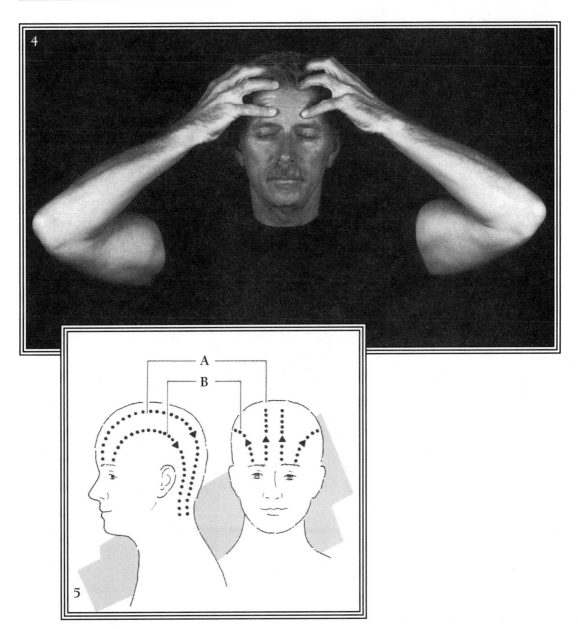

4. Fingers apart, grip your head and work along parallel and diagonal lines extending over the top of your head and down your neck (**5A, 5B**).

6. Draw soft circles on your temples (no pressure).

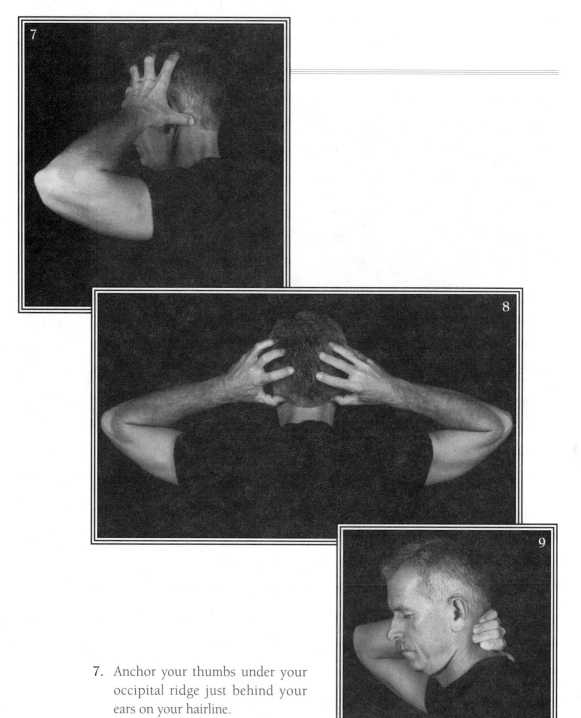

7. Anchor your thumbs under your occipital ridge just behind your ears on your hairline.
8. Tilt your head forward and back.
9. Squeeze the back of your neck.

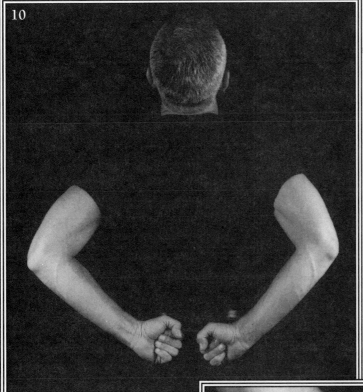

10. Bunch your fists against your sacrum and lean back, or lie down on the floor and place a tennis ball under your sacrum.

11. Pinch your little toe (and your big toe).

If your headache is raging, just try 9, 10, 11.

C. CONGESTION FROM COLDS, ALLERGIES, AND SINUSITIS

There seems to be an increase in the number of people (on both sides of the Atlantic) complaining of congestion and allergies. Damage to the ozone layer and the increase of toxic pollutants are major factors. But weather conditions, pollen and mold, infection or inflammation can all bung up nose and head and make our eyes stream and our lives miserable. A new term, "Sick Building Syndrome," has been coined to describe allergies related to unhealthy substances (anything from pigeon droppings to mold) circulated via a building's heating and cooling systems.

As with headaches, it's useful to note the times and seasonal or dietary factors contributing to the attacks to get some sort of a hold on what's going on as well as to establish links and patterns. Chiropractic physician Dr. Linda Li of New York and Boulder, Colorado uses kinesiology (muscle testing) to help track the source of allergies, with some fascinating results. One of her patients came regularly each Monday with terrible allergies, so she asked the woman about her Sunday activities.

"Nothing very exciting," the patient shrugged. "Mainly housecleaning." Dr. Li checked out her reactions to different cleaning products and discovered she was allergic to ammonia.

Perhaps you suddenly develop allergies after moving to a new neighborhood or new town. It's worthwhile finding out what toxic fumes you're exposed to from local factories or toxic waste dumps. But you could also be allergic to the synthetic fibers of your newly installed carpeting or curtains. If you have an old refrigerator, make sure it isn't emitting toxic fumes. Check windows or ventilators for mold. Ask locally about pollen counts or other allergy-inducing substances in the air.

Secondhand smoke in your home and office can also cause allergies, asthma, and other breathing difficulties for you and especially for your children. BBC-TV's *Horizon* series documented current studies relating secondhand smoke to a range of problems, from allergies to lung cancer, in "Smokers Can Harm Your Health" in 1992 (first aired on PBS in the U.S. on February 1, 1994). Women exposed to secondhand smoke risk a 30 to 50 percent chance of developing lung cancer, according to an American Medical Association report (*AMA Journal*, June 8, 1994). The U.S. Environmental Protection Agency blames secondhand smoke for 3,000 lung cancer deaths and 53,000 heart disease deaths in nonsmokers each year (*New York Times*, June 17, 1994).

Unfortunately, Germany does not share the zeal of Britain and North America for raising consciousness about smoking-related diseases, or for increasing restrictions on smoking in public places. Excessive smoking, especially among young Germans, makes smoke-filled but poorly ventilated cafés and restaurants a nightmare for nonsmokers.

Outdated factories, emissions from "Trabi" cars, and random toxic waste dumping in former East Germany created appalling breathing conditions that have eased a lot since 1989. I remember driving from Berlin to Dresden in 1990 with a handkerchief over my mouth and nose, eyes streaming from the sulfurous haze. I felt saddened by the long-term effect of such pollution on the lungs of newborn babes and the food chain.

Mexico City, Los Angeles, and Tokyo are equally heavily polluted cities.

Incessant winter rains combined with inhuman living conditions and air pollution from coal or paraffin fires in Cape Town's most densely populated areas not only contribute to some of the highest TB rates in the world but to an abnormally high incidence of breathing problems—especially asthma—in young children. It was encouraging to receive positive feedback from mothers who learned some shiatsu techniques and then taught their asthmatic kids how to help themselves breathe more easily.

While posing for the photos for joggers in this guide, Patty Horii, a fourth-generation Japanese-American from San Francisco, told me about the yai-to technique her grandfather used successfully for years to help her brother through asthma attacks. He would take a piece of string and measure the circumference of the boy's right foot (left for girls). He would then tie a knot in the string, place it around the boy's neck just under the Adam's apple, pull the knot down to the right of the spine (left for girls), and burn moxa (mugwort) on that point three or four times, for three or four days. You need to be properly trained to use moxa, so please don't try, but you might achieve the same result by lighting a stick of incense and holding it close to that point. Don't touch the skin. If the point gets too hot, move the stick away a little (see diagram on p. 28).

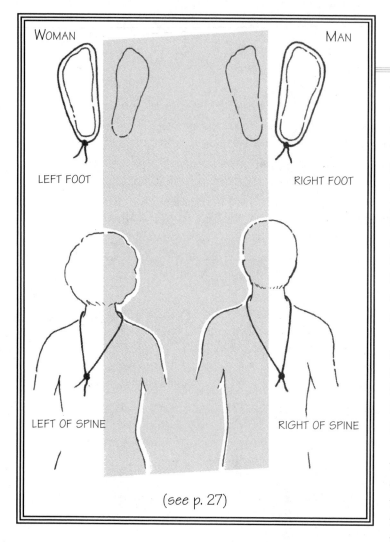

WOMAN

LEFT FOOT

MAN

RIGHT FOOT

LEFT OF SPINE

RIGHT OF SPINE

(see p. 27)

The sudden and seemingly unexplained onset of allergies can also imply a gradual weakening of the immune system, and should be checked immediately by a physician. I remember suddenly developing allergies to cat hair, dust, and MSG (used in some Chinese restaurants) in New York City just a year or so before my cancer was diagnosed.

Tests on my body before surgery showed a high lead content, which is not surprising considering the years I lived in New York City and London.

Through conscious effort we can control some of our environmental factors, but not all. Experts advise drinking bottled water and following a diet high in vegetables, B complex vitamins, vitamin C, and garlic, and low in dairy, wheat, corn, and other mucus-stimulating foods. Native American healers advise echinacea (to boost immune system), ginger tea, inhaling vapor from infused eucalyptus leaves, or cleansing the air by burning sage leaves. Some people chew on vitamin C tablets to ward off an allergy attack, some swear by hot, spicy foods (Mexican or Indian) to decongest, others work out at gyms, while those less fortunate must rely heavily on medications just to get through a working day. Anyone suffering from allergies and/or sinus problems knows how stress and tiredness can weaken resistance.

Whatever the extent of your problem, you might find relief by trying a few key shiatsu exercises. Again, they will be most effective if you use them as prevention or when the symptoms first hit you.

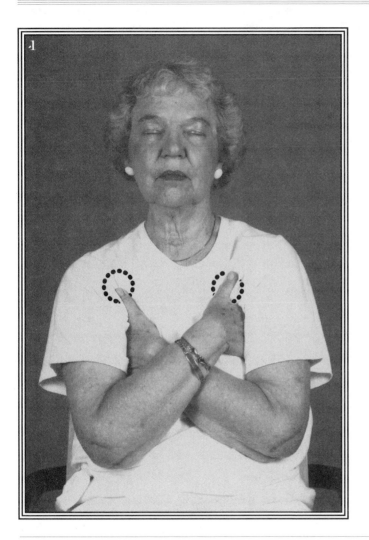

Anti-Congestion Exercises

1. Slide your hand under your armpit and squeeze your arm against it. Extend
   your thumb and press in firmly. Press points around a circle between shoulder
   and collarbone. (I learned this exercise by chance from Linda Clarke, an asthma
   sufferer who knew nothing about shiatsu. She did this instinctively to help her
   exhale during an attack, without knowing she was activating the meridian associated with the lungs and the intake of fresh ki into the body.)

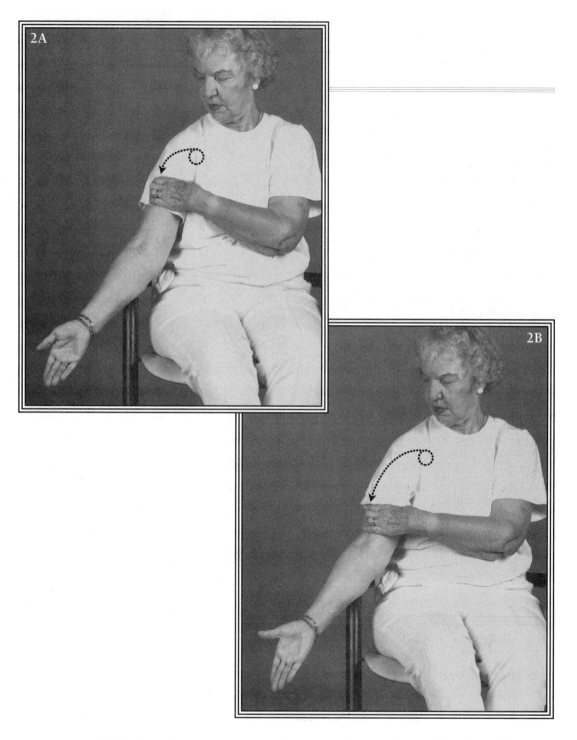

2A–D. Stretch out your arm, palm up, and press along a line from the circle between collarbone and shoulder to your thumb.

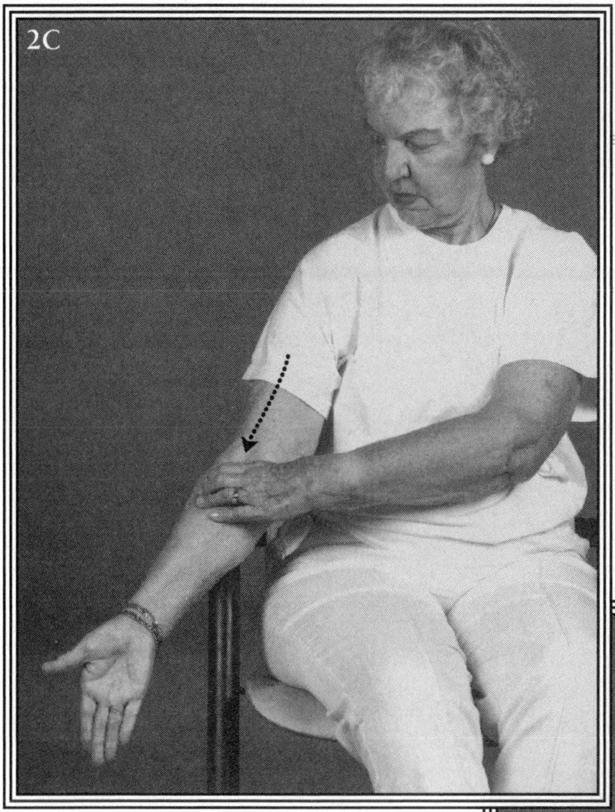
2C

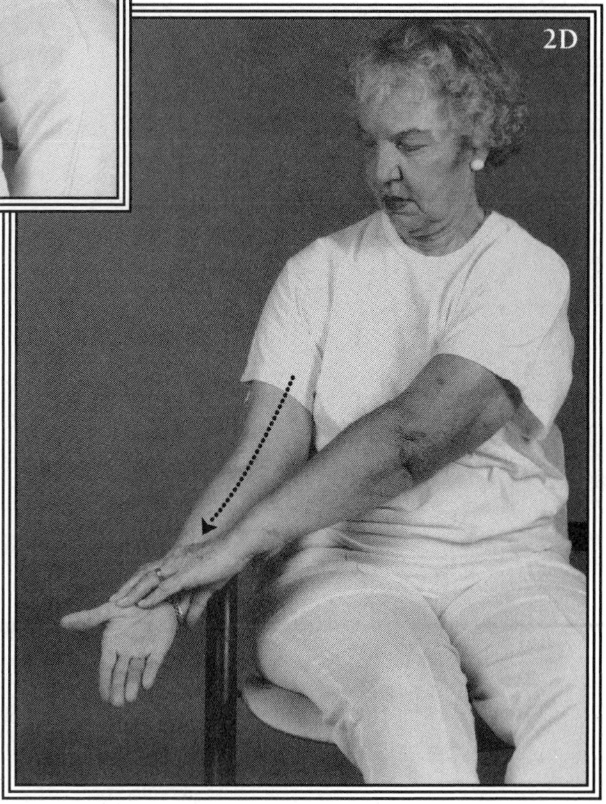
2D

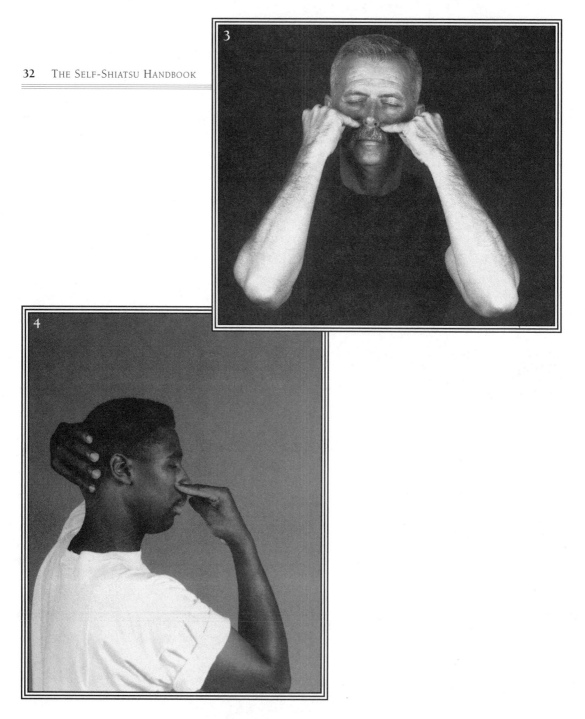

3. Press points on either side of your nostrils.
4. Press nostril points and points just below the first cervical vertebra, simultaneously.

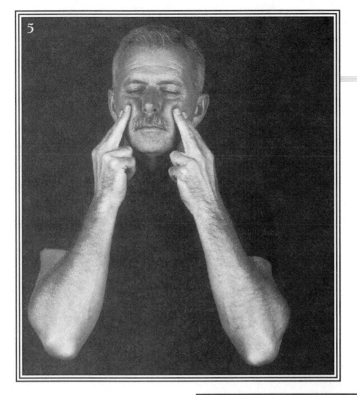

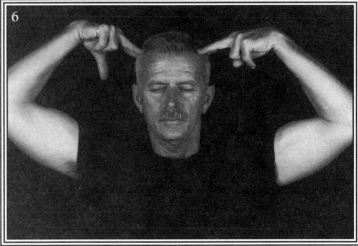

5. Press under your cheekbones with two fingers.
6. Make Vs of your fingers and
press the sides of your head
to ease sinus pain. Try different points to discover
which ones ease your pain.
7. To drain sinus congestion utilizing the pull of gravity, hang
down over a chair arm or the edge of your bed.
8. Try the headache sequence.

Again, as with the headache sequence, don't be in a hurry. Press in and release
slowly and gently.

D. CONSTIPATION

A student of mine in Hamburg once summed up the "three white vices" of Western civilization that cause constipation: white, upright toilets, white sugar, and white flour.

Those of us who've traveled in the Orient well know what it's like to squat over a small hole. Primitive, maybe, but the squat is nature's most practical way of stimulating a bowel movement. If you're a constipation sufferer and can't manage to squat, you can modify the squat stretch when you are sitting on the toilet, by raising your feet and clasping your knees or by placing your feet on a footstool.

Climb stairs every day. If you live in a hilly city (Zürich, Cape Town, San Francisco), make good use of the landscape: walk uphill as much as you can.

In my classes constipation sufferers often relate their problems to a severe upbringing and military-style toilet training.

One New Yorker told me she had developed such an inhibition as a kid that at fifty-five she still needed a stack of magazines beside the toilet to read to help pass the time. She raised her own four kids without rules about "potty time" and they grew up without any constipation problems whatsoever.

The experts again advise plenty of bottled water, fresh fruit, veggies, and whole grains to clear and move the system. Meat, especially red meat, can linger uncomfortably in the intestines. One chronic constipation sufferer swears by a morning glass of whole fruit chunks tossed in a blender as being far more effective than plain fruit juice. I have heard people from Zürich to Bombay to Cape Town praise fennel tea as a wonderful remedy. Many Indian restaurants have bowls of fennel seeds for you to chew at the end of your meal as a digestion aid. Vegetarians rarely have problems with constipation.

Travel, a sudden change of diet, stress, or a crowded schedule can all throw you off balance. But whether constipation is a chronic or an occasional problem, give the following exercises a try.

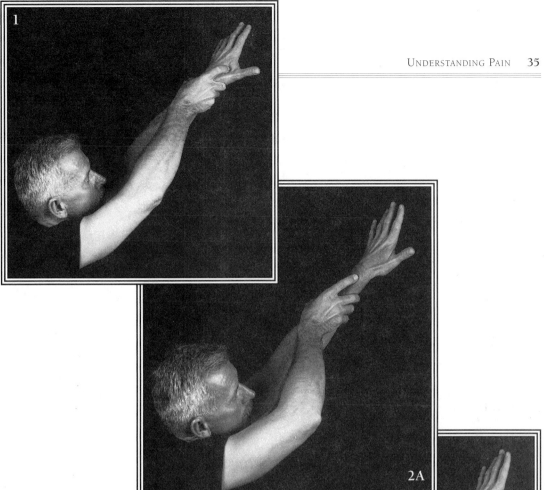

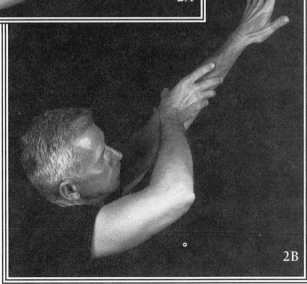

Anti-Constipation Exercises

1. Raise your arm and press the point at the top of the triangle between thumb and first finger. This is one of the best remedies for constipation. Get to know it well. Press it as often as you can.

2A, 2B. Continue pressing down in a line from that point along the outside of your arm all the way to your shoulder.

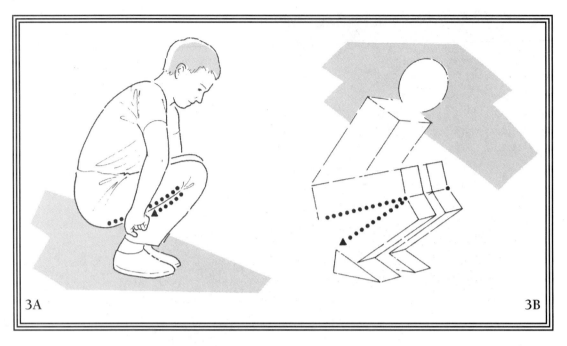

3A

3B

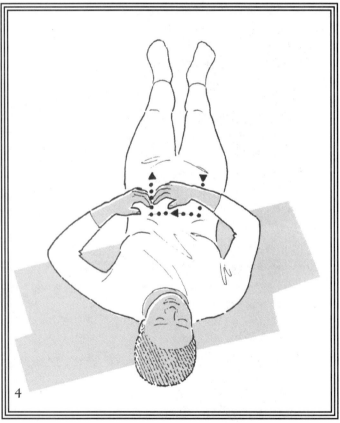

4

3. Sit in a squat. Imagine your leg is square (**3A**). Bunch your fists against the outer edge of your thighs and work down from top of thigh to ankle (**3B**).

4. Lie down on a comfortable mat. Do self-shiatsu around your large intestine. Using your fingertips, work in soft circular movements up the ascending colon on the right-hand side, across the transverse, and down the descending colon.

E. INDIGESTION

Make sure you aren't eating too quickly, or eating while walking, driving, or on the telephone, like a typical New Yorker! Chew well. Chew fennel seeds after eating, or sip peppermint or chamomile tea. If you have problems with gas, eat oranges for dessert.

For all forms of intestinal discomfort, or to combat that bloated feeling, try the anti-constipation exercises. Also try tapping your breastbone. Try pressing points about an inch on either side of your navel.

In my workshops, when students who happen to be health practitioners ask me for advice about a patient who suffers from problems with digestion, I suggest they share a meal with that person and observe his or her behavior around food. And ask if he or she grew up in a family where everyone fought at mealtimes or scrambled for food. A family history of discordant dinners can often result in chronic problems with digestion in adulthood.

F. BACK PAIN

I believe we have all experienced back pain at some time in our lives and sought different remedies to conquer it, ranging from surgery to painkillers to ice packs to heating pads, and from $3 jars of Tiger Balm to $3,000 vibrating armchairs. According to the *Visual Encyclopedia of Natural Healing*, back pain is the major cause of disability in Americans under the age of forty-five.

Being deskbound can exacerbate back pain, especially if you're stuck behind a computer keyboard. Being a couch potato is even worse.

When I ruptured a disc in London in the late 1960s, while working as an industrial journalist on *The Times*, a chiropractor recommended swimming as one of the best ways to combat back problems. I have followed his advice ever since, with no recurring disc problems. The Florida Back Institute at Boca Raton has discovered that people who suffer chronic pain after undergoing low-back surgery find relief, for hours or days, after swimming around with dolphins (*Fort Lauderdale Sun-Sentinel*, June 30, 1994). Dolphin Research Team Director Beth Smart is currently conducting before and after blood checks on the patients to determine chemical changes—especially increased levels of endorphins—after each swim.

Smart describes the dolphins as semi-captive and untrained, as they swim voluntarily into an enclosed area of Key Largo, Florida, where the experiments take place. There is no physical contact between patient and dolphin, but she says dolphins are friendlier toward some patients than toward others. Patients claim the experience gives them greater and more sustained relief than standard forms of swimming therapy and conventional treatment. Some are experiencing relief for the first time after twenty years of chronic pain. Perhaps the joyful experience helps raise endorphin levels. Or perhaps the "vibes" dolphins emit are a potent form of ki.

The study, while still in the early stages, confirms my belief that joy is a healing tool.

Even if you don't have access to dolphins, you'll find swimming a relief. Swimming exercises the whole body and is a great way to release back tension, especially after traveling long distances (road or rail). The baby pose of hatha yoga (where you crouch down on all fours) is also a great way to relieve back problems.

As the daughter of a Cornishwoman, I was fascinated to discover a sacred site for back pain sufferers at an ancient formation of rocks known as Men-An-Tol, Penwith, on the way to Land's End at Cornwall's southwest tip. Men-An-Tol typifies this land of myths and legends and sacred Celtic sites. It's far from the nearest hamlet and you have to approach it through the fields on foot.

Men-An-Tol means "stone with a hole" in the Cornish language, and such is the central donut-like stone, flanked on either side by two phallic stones. As the legend goes, climb through the hole nine times and your back pains are over. Actually, the legend makes sense. Climbing through the tight hole involves crawling and stretching arms and legs alternately, surely one of the best practical remedies for lower back pain (see p. 42).

You can create your own Men-An-Tol by hanging up an old car tire in your backyard, not just for your kids to use as a swing, but for you to climb through a few times a day. Failing this, plop down to all fours as often as you can. Make good use of the crawl, alternately stretching your arms and legs.

One of my students in Dresden told me about a farmer near the Czech border who eased his back pain by moving his upper body from left to right in slow, graceful movements, as though cutting tall grass with a scythe. Others find relief in the fish pose of yoga (or by placing a cushion under the upper back) or by sleeping with their knees resting on a pile of cushions.

Most standard forms of back pain are caused by poor lifting habits, sitting in one position for too long, or lack of exercise. Monitor your back pain for any recurring patterns. If you experience pain at the end of the day, examine your work environment for sources of stress, like a desk that's too high or a chair that's too low, instruments you have problems reaching or operating, or objects that are cumbersome for you to move. If you use a computer, read the "Computer Workers" section in Part II (pp. 69–75).

Make sure you have comfortable shoes, especially if you walk to and from work. High heels, narrow, or flimsy fashionable shoes can all cause back pain. This is plain common sense, but we seldom notice the obvious, the familiar, until a problem arises.

Back pain can also be caused by emotional stress, poor digestion, or menstrual problems.

Sudden or acute back pain could be the symptom of a range of less obvious but serious medical problems (like lung or kidney disease) requiring professional diagnosis and treatment. So be aware of all the possibilities.

If you suffer from occasional back pain, become more prevention-conscious. Stretch several times a day. Make sure there's some support for your lower back when you work at a desk. Exercise in your chair, by moving your feet up and down and drawing circles with your hips. Weave a few exercises into your working day, or stretch each time you get up to go to the bathroom.

If hatha yoga is too extreme, try swimming, tai chi, or a gym to help build muscle flexibility and strength.

Some years ago, a married couple in London asked me to give them shiatsu, as both of them suffered from back pain, especially in the morning. I walked into their bedroom and examined their mattress. It was soft and lumpy.

"Buy yourselves a decent mattress or futon," I suggested. They did, and noticed an immediate improvement after a night's sleep.

In my years of working with shiatsu in different countries I have seen back pain eased by acupuncture, reflexology, shiatsu, chiropractic deep muscle work combined with manipulation, ear acupuncture combined with manipulation, and qi gong, where the practitioner doesn't even touch the body. But I have also seen a Thai chef ease a customer's pain in a restaurant by squeezing her neck and shoulders in a simple, instinctive form of shiatsu.

Often it is the intuition of the practitioner and the way he or she determines the subtle origin of the problem that is the key factor. A word, a touch, something strikes a familiar chord and the back is harmonized.

I have heard a spine adjust itself during meditation, when the person was sitting perfectly still. We explain this as a clear movement of ki, quickened by concentration and deep breathing.

Sometimes back pain defies all theories and methods, including expensive surgery and advanced medical procedures. On July 14, 1994, the *New England Journal of Medicine* reported a study done by Hoag Memorial Hospital in Newport Beach, California, showing that advanced magnetic resonance imaging (MRI) can often lead to unnecessary surgery because physicians wrongly assume that spinal abnormalities and degenerated discs cause back pain. In the control study on a number of men and women without back pain, research radiologist Dr. Michael N. Brant-Zawadzki discovered that most of them had an array of spinal abnormalities, including herniated and degenerated discs.

Back specialists at other medical centers have come to similar conclusions, throwing diagnoses and treatment into a hot area of debate. "Most back pain is never explained," admits Dr. Robert Boyd, orthopedic surgeon at Massachusetts General Hospital in Boston (*New York Times*, July 14, 1994).

Someone versed in oriental medicine would challenge Dr. Boyd by offering diagnoses related to energy imbalances in the meridian system.

Seek second or third opinions on your back problems. And start a fitness routine for your back. Don't stress or force anything, though. Select only those of the following exercises that feel comfortable for you.

Anti-Back Pain Exercises

1. Here's a simple exercise to try if you are plagued by pain. If you can't manage a lotus or half-lotus, sit comfortably or lie down. Now, as you inhale, imagine an elevator moving up inside your spine, vertebra by vertebra. Visualize it as one of those clear structures you see on high-tech buildings. As it moves up slowly, feel it dissolving pain and tension. See it ascend through the top of your head, then descend and start again at your coccyx, if necessary.

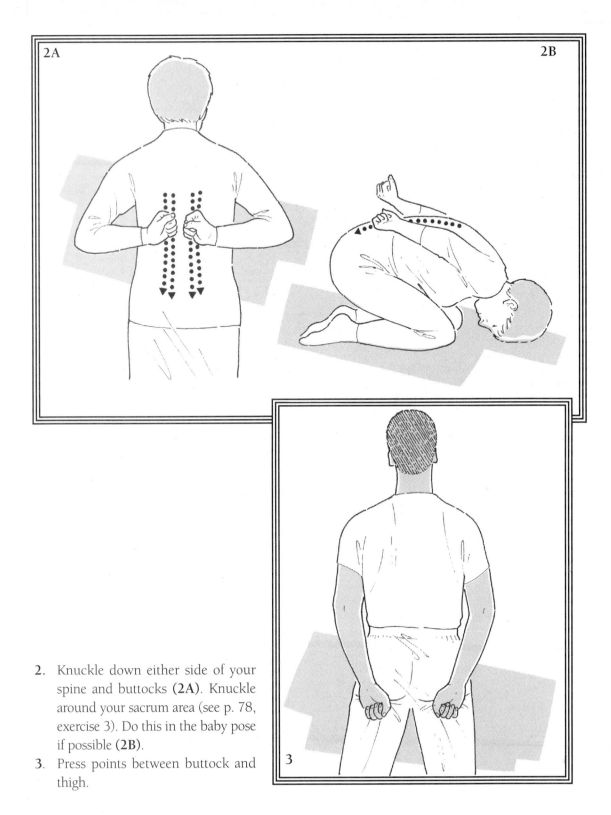

2. Knuckle down either side of your spine and buttocks (**2A**). Knuckle around your sacrum area (see p. 78, exercise 3). Do this in the baby pose if possible (**2B**).

3. Press points between buttock and thigh.

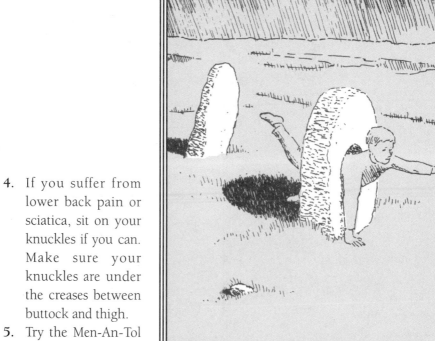

4. If you suffer from lower back pain or sciatica, sit on your knuckles if you can. Make sure your knuckles are under the creases between buttock and thigh.

5. Try the Men-An-Tol stretch (see p. 38).

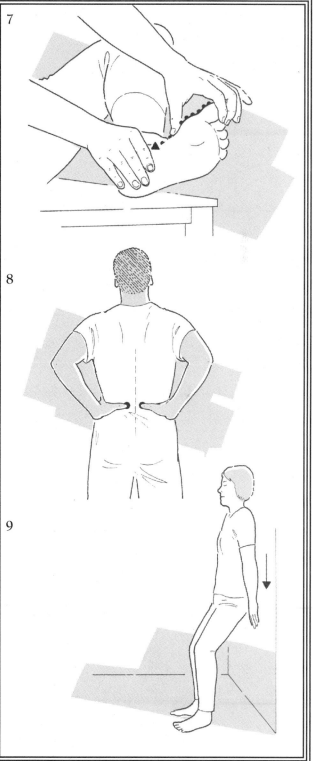

6. Pinch your Achilles tendon (see p. 79).
7. Work your thumb along your instep from toe to heel.
8. Press points on either side of your spine directly opposite your navel.
9. Press your back against a wall. Bend your knees if you can, but don't do this if it feels uncomfortable.
10. Lie flat on the floor. Inhale and tense every muscle. Then exhale and slowly release face, shoulders, arms, hands, back, buttocks, legs, feet.

Again, select the easiest exercises first, or those you most enjoy, and work them into your day. Don't feel you have to achieve all of the exercises—you don't. Also arrange a sequence to suit you.

G. INSOMNIA

If counting sheep doesn't help you, and you are weary of making yourself hot drinks with honey, watching TV, listening to music, reading, or doing your taxes, you could try some of the following exercises.

1. Lie faceup. Slide your fingers under your neck and apply gentle pressure.

2. Rest the fingers of one hand on the palm of the other hand, thumb just below wrist.

3. Do deep breathing. Visualize the breath as a silver stream entering your left nostril, sitting at the top of your nose as you hold your breath to a count of five, and exiting your right nostril. Repeat.

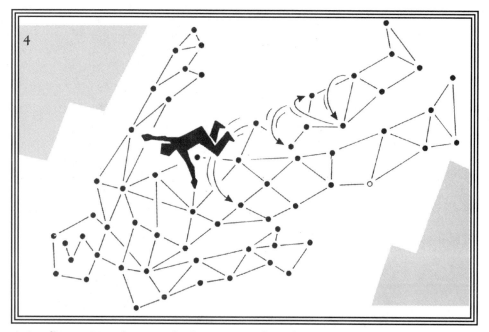

4. Lie faceup. Visualize your body as a complex of points and lines. Imagine yourself as a tiny figure jumping and zigzagging its way from point to point, from left to right, starting with your big toes and continuing to the top of your head. You'll probably fall asleep before you get halfway.

5. Tighten your entire body, from the tips of your toes to your scalp. Release each part in turn.

H. "THE BLUES" AND LOW ENERGY

There are no simple, immediate cures here, but regular exercise helps to prevent and ease the problem—it's hard to feel blue or low after a good walk or bicycle ride. Cut down on sugar, caffeine, nicotine, and alcohol, to avoid highs and lows. Other useful tips:

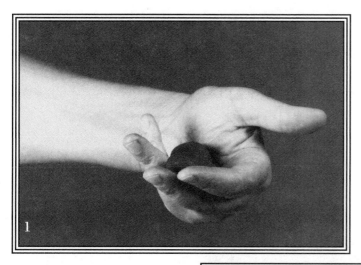

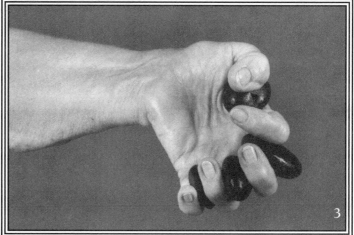

1. Take a handful of pebbles, roll them around in your palm, and squeeze them.
2. Open and close your hand several times.
3. Now squeeze the pebbles between your fingers.

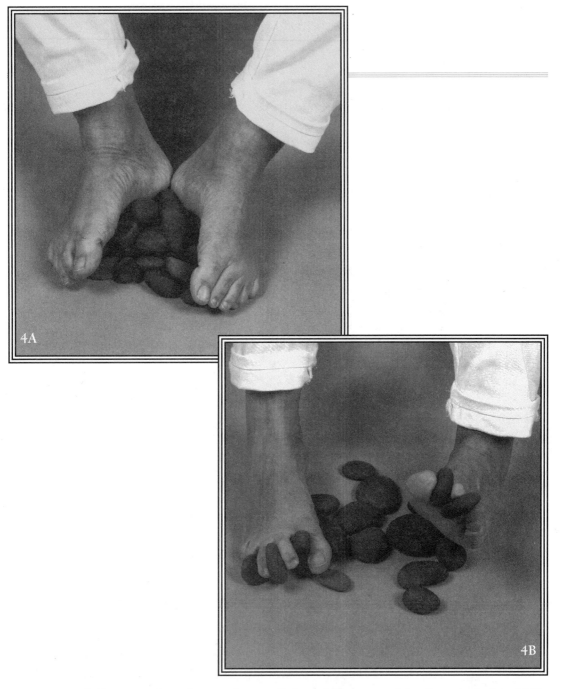

4A

4B

4. Press your bare feet on them, roll the pebbles around the floor underfoot (**4A**), and try picking them up between your toes (**4B**). You're using the pebbles as a speedy form of self-shiatsu. Feet and hands are like the keyboards of the body, a quick way of accessing your entire energy system.

Choose a variety of pebbles, knobbly, smooth, large, small, whatever feels good for you. I come from mining families (on both sides) and so grew up with a deep love of stones and a sensitivity to their different vibrations.

I collect stones on my travels and keep them in a jar on my desk as a paperweight to connect me with the rest of the world. During breaks from the computer, I squeeze them in my hands or underfoot as a quick pick-me-up or when I hit creative snags.

You may prefer to use just one favorite pebble—even a squash or tennis ball. "Pebble therapy" is also good for poor circulation, or for stiff joints, or as rehabilitation to keep energy moving in the rest of the body when you are recovering from surgery or a damaged limb.

WOMEN'S CORNER

========

I. MENSTRUAL PAIN

Most girls and women—of all cultures—experience menstrual pain at some time in their lives. Some suffer so badly they miss school or work for a couple of days each month. Some experience a slight pain or discomfort that is eased by exercise or a hot water bottle or, in some cases, by eating hot food. Throughout the generations, women have worked out dozens of different remedies for themselves, from herbal concoctions to compresses.

Some experience sharp abdominal pains or lower back pains or both. Some women suffer the worst symptoms of PMT (premenstrual tension), but no physical pain. I recall a doctor telling two school friends of mine that their "bad cramps" would ease as soon as they married and "produced children" but until then they just had to accept their pain. Both continued to have cramps after they married and had children.

Women who switch to vegetarian diets often notice a marked difference, fewer cramps and a much lighter flow. Women who cut out meat and dairy products just before menstruating have also experienced less painful periods. Many find it helpful to drink veggie juices, especially a combination of carrot, parsley, and beet juice, just before menstruation. Those who crave sugar (especially chocolate) find it useful to take B complex or calcium supplements.

Regular exercise is a vitally important way of counteracting those "sluggish" or painful days.

During my travels, I make a note of remedies that seem to transcend particular cultures: red raspberry leaf tea for heavy periods or cramps; chamomile tea for a late period; peppermint or spearmint tea for light periods.

Shamaan Ochaum of Austin, Texas, a medicine woman of Native American, African, and Irish heritage, describes both menstruation and menopause as sacred and powerful transitions according to traditional Native American beliefs. Among the Apache, the onset of menstruation is seen as a time when a girl becomes intensely psychic, and a channel for healing.

For painful periods she recommends passion flower, red raspberry leaves, and skullcap; for heavy periods she suggests plantain, black cohosh, and chaste tree berry.

More and more women and girls are seeking ancient rituals as a way of celebrating their cycles, to break the "curse" image of our Western upbringing. Some organize nature retreats, or fertility dances on beaches, among trees, or in the mountains, giving themselves time and space to "vision-quest" or explore their heightened awareness during menstruation.

Upstate New York herbalist Susun Weed claims many women reduce their menstrual cramps or PMS symptoms by "honoring their moontime." Her findings are supported by Yarmouth, Maine, gynecologist Christine Northrup, who traces most female troubles to the sense of shame many girls experience at menarche ("Blood Sisters," *New Age Journal*, June 1994).

Many women gain insight into cycles of pain and tension by keeping journals and tracing patterns month by month, an equally useful way of familiarizing themselves with the ebb and flow of moods and emissions and fertile days. Obviously the more in tune women are with their cycle and bodily rhythms, the closer they are to self-healing. Shiatsu exercises fit in well with this theory as a form of prevention against pain or discomfort, either midmonth or a couple of days before menstruation begins.

Some of you may already practice simple versions of the exercises listed below without realizing the shiatsu connection. A Swiss (part Iranian) student of mine told me she used to ask her mother to press the inside of her legs when she had cramps as a teenager, one of our key shiatsu zones for menstrual problems!

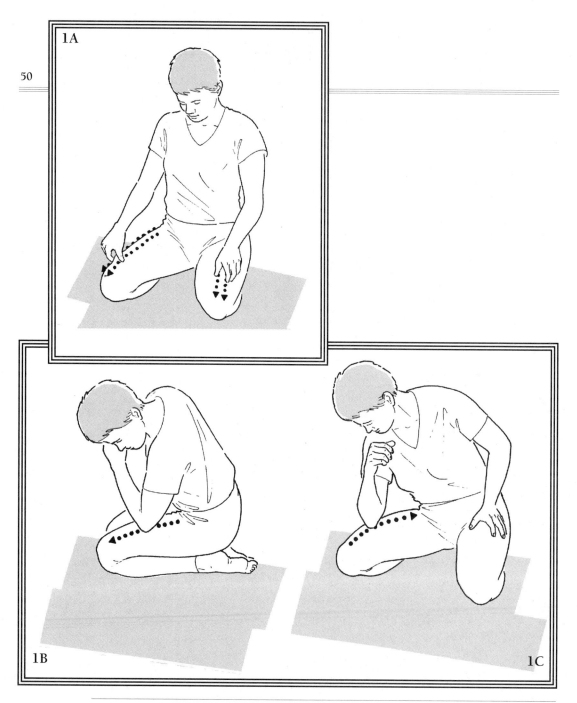

Exercises Against Menstrual Pain

1. Kneel down. Pinch your thighs (**1A**). Elbow down the outside line (**1B**) and up the inside (**1C**).

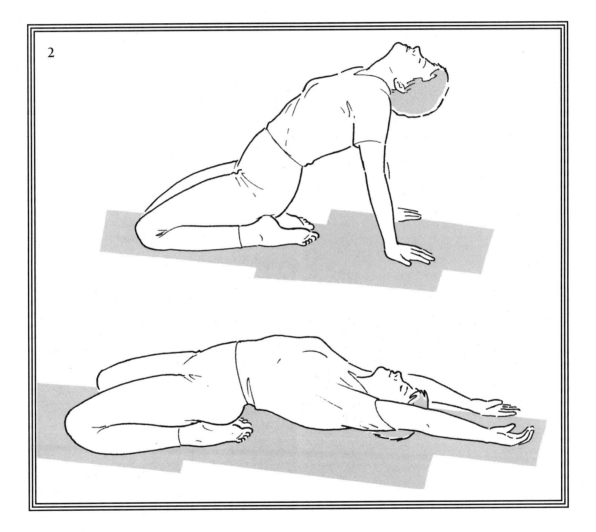

2. Lean back and place your hands behind you. If you can, lean on your elbows or lower your back to the floor. But don't force it; don't stress your lower back.

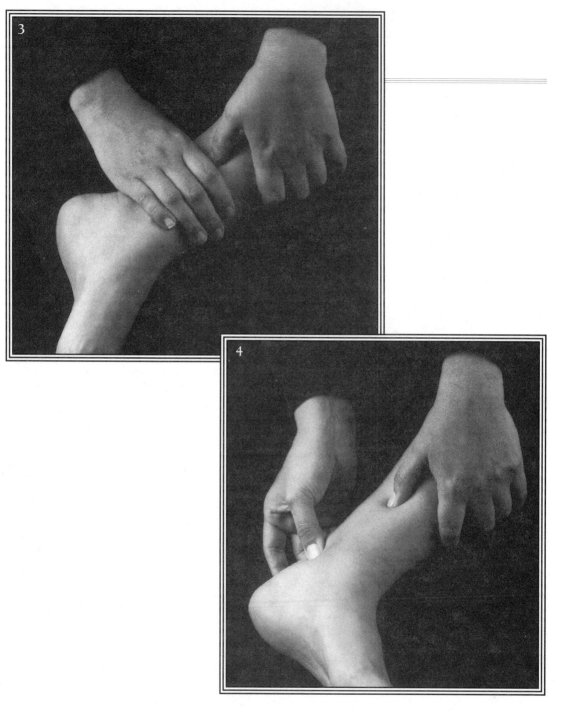

3. Press a point on the inside of your leg, four finger widths up from your ankle. The point is often sensitive or painful.
4. Press the above point and Achilles tendon simultaneously.

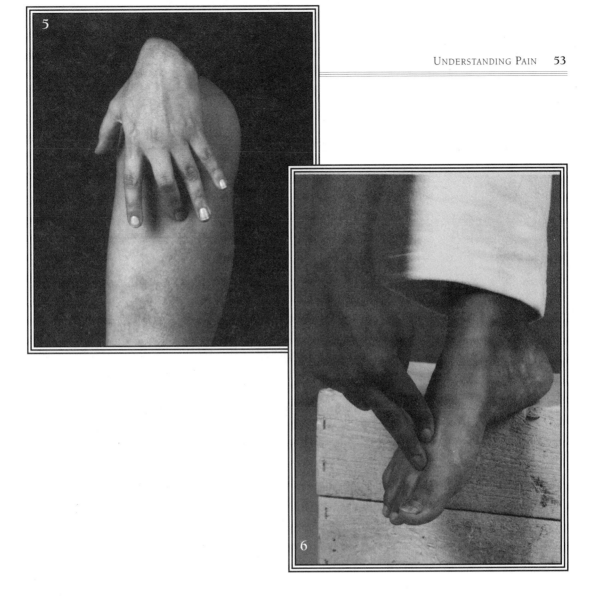

5. Place your hand on top of your bended knee. Swivel your middle finger to a point outside your shinbone.

6. Make a V and press points between your big toe and second toe.

• If your period is late, press the points hard and fast, especially 3. But avoid these points, especially 3, during pregnancy. Also see p. 108.

• See the section on family shiatsu for exercises you can do with your partner or friend to beat menstrual pain.

J. MENOPAUSE

According to Native American belief, menopause is a sacred time for a woman. She is free of her childbearing/child-rearing years and revered for her quickening power and insight. Rituals and ceremonies celebrate this rite of passage. "They dance around her with juniper and sage," says medicine woman Shamaan Ochaum. "She becomes an elder and seer, and is released from many of her duties as a caretaker." Germaine Greer, in her excellent work *The Change—Women, Aging and the Menopause*, describes the black garb of older Mediterranean women as a similar rite of passage symbolizing new privileges and the space and time for women to go off on their own, explore, sit with friends, travel. "Poets since classical times have celebrated an ideal stage of tranquil thoughtfulness to round off a busy life," Greer says.

We need to remind ourselves of such ancient rituals when we confront the menopausal myths and misconceptions of our own societies: the music hall jokes, the negative media image of older women compared with older men, prompting some women to race into plastic surgery for solutions.

Many of the great feminist writers of the 1960s and 1970s such as Greer are experiencing their own "climacteric" and are opening windows on the subject in refreshing political and medical analyses. They challenge the taboos and dispel the obsession with hormone replacement therapy that dominates most books on menopause.

In the United States some 43 million women are menopausal or post-menopausal, and the number increases by about half a million women a year, according to *Menopause, the Silent Passage*, by Gail Sheehy. Yet the subject is still gripped by a "shocking breadth of ignorance and denial," as she writes. Support groups are sprouting all over the country where women gather to share this natural experience for which most of them are totally unprepared and badly misinformed.

Many baby boomers undergoing menopause in the 1980s and 1990s talk about the subject in a way that was absolutely taboo for our mothers' and grandmothers' generations, and alas, continues to be taboo for many of our contemporaries. Some women continue to suffer in silence and think they are going mad, while others experience no discomfort at all and wonder what the fuss is about.

During a group discussion on PBS even a gynecologist admitted she didn't recognize her own first "hot flash" one night, and went off the next day to buy a lighter-weight cover for her bed!

When I experienced my own first hot flash (or "hot flush" as it is more accurately described in England), I thought my house was on fire. I jumped out of bed and rushed around sniffing for the smoke until I realized the raging heat was internal. American feminists have swapped the term "hot flashes" for "power surges," an interesting subconscious recognition of the rite of passage celebrated by ancient societies.

Medical texts differ on the causes. But it's generally believed hot flashes are prompted by mixed signals in the body. At the onset of menopause, the luteinizing hormone (LH), which helps trigger ovulation, surges. But the ovaries say, sorry, the shop's closed, and the LH sets off alarm bells by dilating surface blood vessels.

Without any warning or buildup, we start to sweat profusely and go red in the face. Alcohol, hot, spicy food, and caffeine can be triggering factors. We all handle our power surges in different ways: by wearing loose, layered clothing, so outer layers can be discarded, by rubbing ice on the back of our necks, by sipping ginseng or licorice root tea (natural sources of estrogen) or red raspberry leaf tea.

Some women sail though menopause symptom-free. Others experience the wallop of power surges (night or day), weight increase, mood swings, irritability, memory lapses, tearfulness, vaginal dryness, dry skin and hair loss, paranoia, varicose veins, incontinence, insomnia, depression.

Experts advise vitamins (especially A, C, E, and B complex) and regular physical exercise (yoga, tai chi, walking, weights, cycling) to help modify symptoms and maintain a sense of well-being. Addictive habits (caffeine, alcohol, smoking, etc.) intensify symptoms and should be cut down or cut out. According to some herbalists, the effects of a sluggish liver (and slower metabolism) can be offset by lemon and garlic first thing in the morning or by eating dandelion roots and wild yams. Vitamin E oil and sesame seed oil help dry skin. For a dry vagina or atrophy vaginitis, doctors advise rubbing one of the following in the vagina: vitamin E oil, aloe vera, or a commercial gel, *Rosmarinus Prunus* (the latter, a Wala product, might be available only in Europe). The most natural way of obtaining aloe vera is to keep a plant in your home, snap a stem, and use the sticky substance directly. Aloe vera is also a wonderful remedy for dry skin and for burns.

For bladder incontinence, you can strengthen your muscles by alternately tightening and releasing the vagina at any time during the day, or practice the stop-go technique during urination.

Weight-bearing exercises (weight lifting, walking, jogging) and calcium-rich (but low-fat) foods help maintain bone density and prevent weight gain. Fears of osteoporosis and heart attacks send many women racing for hormone replacement therapy, without exploring their options, and this underlines the controversial core of the whole subject.

Those of us with a history of breast cancer, in ourselves or our families, cannot receive HRT, because estrogen feeds breast cancer cells. The optimum time for breast cancer is at the onset of menopause, when estrogen surges in the body. My own belief in taking calcium over HRT inspired me to sign up for a two-year research project at the University of Texas Southwestern Medical Center, on the effects of calcium citrate as an alternative to estrogen to prevent bone density loss. As a vegetarian, I am encouraged by statistics that show we maintain bone density better than meat eaters.

Women who are feeling the extremes of menopause owe it to themselves to research all their options before being rushed into HRT by medical doctors.

The estrogen patch (low dose) can be a compromise solution for many women with a family history of osteoporosis and heart disease, or who find the symptoms of menopause intolerable.

Other women prefer to concentrate on their own input in terms of diet, exercise, meditation, and allowing the "change" to guide them into exploring new studies or creative ventures for themselves. One woman's solution may be wholly inappropriate for another, but either way, an informed choice is the key. Shiatsu, acupuncture, and classical massage can all help to harmonize extreme symptoms.

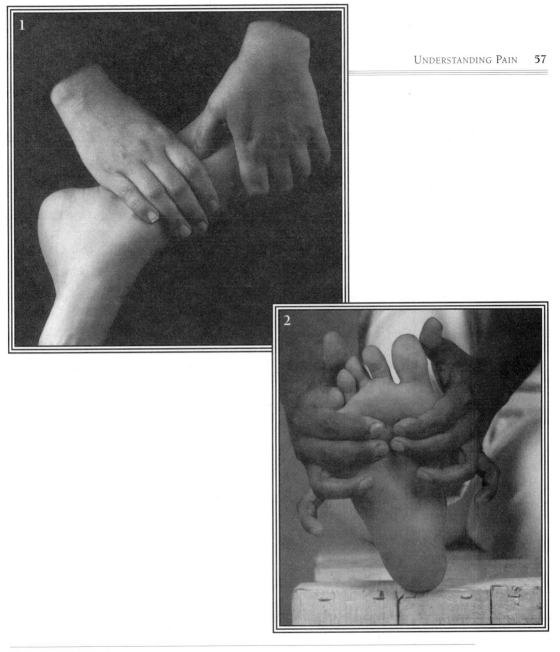

Exercises for Menopause

Follow all the exercises for menstrual pain, and especially:

1. The point four finger widths up from the anklebone is a wonderful way of soothing an intense "power surge" and giving you some control over it.
2. The point under the ball of your foot is also a great help.

K. BREAST HEALTH AND BREAST CANCER

Ironically, it was only after experiencing breast cancer that I gave any serious thought to breast health. As girls, we grow up bombarded by pinup photos and ads of busty women selling everything from car tires to vacations in Africa. But who spoke to us about breast health?

During my teenage years in Cape Town in the late 1950s and early 1960s, it was the Marilyn Monroe look, tight sweaters and high, pointed bras. During my time in London from the mid-1960s to the mid-1970s, it was the flat-chested Twiggy or Mary Quant look. When I returned to North America in the late seventies, it was the braless look and marching topless at protests. But who spoke about breast health?

Most women grow up with misgivings about their breasts, feeling less than the ideal look of the day. In the United States, prior to the 1991–92 government hearings and restrictions on silicone implants following the horror stories about side effects, the ratio of women who sought silicone for breast enlargement, compared with postmastectomy women, was 80:20.

In Britain the ratio was 20:80, the exact opposite.

After my mastectomy in 1987 I joined an increasing number of women who refuse reconstruction surgery or a prosthesis as a quiet way of showing other women (especially in saunas, gyms, and swimming pools) that there can be exercise, health, and life after breast cancer. We buck the myths and, I hope, help to ease fear and ignorance. We're also utilizing our experience to spread information about breast health and breast cancer to prod the government to increase spending on research.

The breast swings like a pendulum between positive and negative images: a symbol of life, nurturing, motherhood, womanhood, and a much-exploited sex symbol and topic of locker room jokes.

But who speaks to us of breast health and exercises or activities as a prevention against breast disease? We owe it to our younger sisters, daughters, and nieces to talk about such things, not only for health but for an inner connection between breast and self that transcends media images or the pop look of the day.

I see the raw end of the topic in postmastectomy classes in hospitals, where many women walk in like apologies for womanhood, holding their arms protectively over their scars as though sheltering injured birds. "Come on, sisters," I say, "raise your arms and stretch them and look up, like a flower opening to the sun.

"Your scars smile when you stretch! Now slowly move your arms up and down like a bird in flight."

A change comes over the room, a release, a feeling of peace. The women begin to lose themselves.

I then teach them the sequence of drawing circles in the air I developed spontaneously after my own mastectomy and practiced every day to Mozart flute and harp concerti.

The art is to draw a larger and larger circle each day; the form offers a simple grid for measuring progress. It is also a graceful and beautiful antidote to the gloom-and-doom image of breast cancer. The "drawing circles" techniques evolved out of my experience of shiatsu and ki exercises.

Within a few weeks of drawing circles I had full extension of my arm and resumed my weekly swimming regimen seven weeks after surgery. I developed no lymph edema (arm swelling), a common postmastectomy problem. I'm certain the exercises, creative visualization, shiatsu, and reflexology all helped me heal much faster than the norm.

I now integrate these exercises with my shiatsu classes, not just to health professionals to teach their own postmastectomy patients, but for everyone to share as a way of raising consciousness about graceful movements to stimulate the flow of energy in breasts and upper body.

In physiological terms the breast is a variation of a sweat gland, a broccoli-like complex of lobes, glands and ducts, and dense connective and adipose tissue. In simpler terms, a milk factory.

Congestion in the circuits can result in all kinds of problems, swelling, and pain prior to menstruation. Breast-feeding is nature's way of activating the circuits, but is no guarantee against breast cancer. Upper body exercises—swimming, weight training, dancing, yoga, tai chi, tennis—are great ways of stimulating the flow of energy in the breasts, to prevent congestion.

Women who experience painful breasts have found regular breast self-massage helpful while soaping themselves under the shower. Similarly, regular self-shiatsu can be useful. Both techniques can also be integrated with self-exams.

Experts like breast surgeon and activist Dr. Susan Love, director of the University of California at Los Angeles (UCLA) Breast Center, advise women to start doing breast self-exams at twenty-five and to have their breasts checked by a physician and an annual mammogram after forty. Opinions on mammography differ on both sides of the Atlantic, and the method, says Dr. Love, isn't 100 percent accurate.

Some lumps (benign or malignant) aren't revealed by mammography, and mammograms can be misread. Women who are wary of X rays can opt for light scans, but only a few hospitals (like the Royal Victoria in Montreal) offer them.

Breast self-knowledge enables women to detect any sudden irregularities or unfamiliar sensations or grains or lumps in the breast or nipple discharge or left/right imbalances—all of which should be checked immediately by a physician. Or two physicians, because lumps can be hard to detect in ropy or dense breast tissue. Of the four doctors who examined my breasts in the months prior to my surgery, two found lumps, two found nothing at all, and I chose to go with the latter, more comforting view, until a fast-growing tumor required immediate surgery. Early detection is not prevention—but it may save your breast.

I urge women to learn from my experience, my activism. Fifty years ago, breast cancer hit 1 in 20 women in the U.S. Today it hits 1 in 8 in the U.S., and I'm told it hits 1 in 13 in Germany. The numbers are increasing globally and including even younger women. Breast cancer activism is a hot political issue in the United States, where women from many different backgrounds, like those who formed the Women's Community Cancer Project of Cambridge, Massachusetts, take to the streets in noisy demonstrations and campaigns to prod the government to increase research funding for causes of breast cancer.

Activism is starting to heat up in Britain but is surprisingly lacking in Germany and Switzerland, even though their rates are among the highest in Europe.

A world map of breast cancer shows the highest incidence in major dairy-producing countries (Germany, Holland, Switzerland, Ireland, New Zealand), which may suggest a high-fat diet is the culprit, or the estrogen they pump into meat and dairy herds. The Orient has the lowest incidence of breast cancer—especially Japan, where a traditional diet is low-fat, nondairy, and high in B complex grains and iodine-rich seaweed and favors fish over meat. But Japanese-American women show the same high rates of breast cancer as other American women, suggesting diet and environmental factors play key roles.

Women in Long Island, New York, where breast cancer rates are abnormally high, were so outraged by inadequate government research locally that they formed a protest group, the 1 in 9 Long Island Breast Cancer Action Group, to study links between breast cancer, toxic waste, polluted water, pesticides, and electromagnetic fields (*New York Times Magazine*, August 15, 1993).

A landmark conference held by the Foundation for a Compassionate Society in Austin, Texas, early in 1994 on the issue of breast cancer and radioactive waste highlighted the increasing vulnerability and incidence of breast cancer among low-income Native, Hispanic, and African-American women in communities close to toxic waste dumps. Generally, the incidence of breast cancer among black women is lower than among white women, but the death rate from breast cancer is much higher among black women.

If a combination of factors, and not just our hereditary genes, causes breast cancer, we owe it to ourselves to strive to maintain breast health, because breasts are rapidly becoming an endangered species.

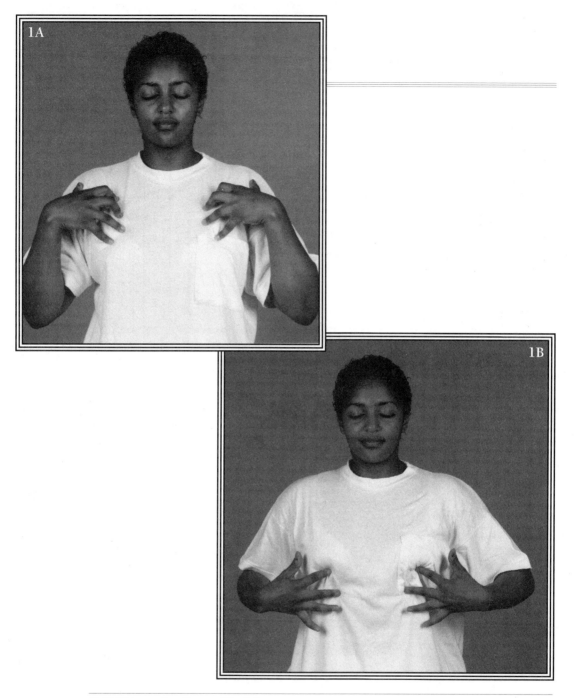

Self-Shiatsu for Breast Health

1. Walk your fingers down vertical lines through your nipples (**1A**) and beyond the breasts (**1B**).

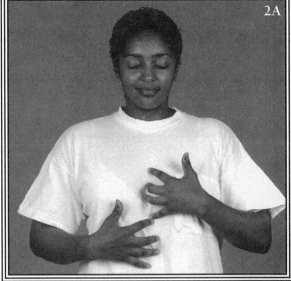

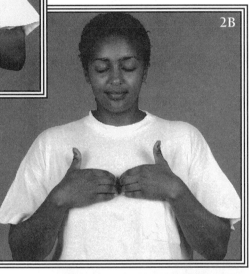

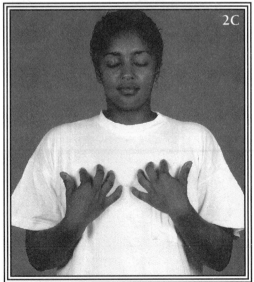

2. Walk your fingers up your sternum (**2A**) to a point between your breasts (**2B**), and then up around the top of your breasts (**2C**).

Integrate the above with breast self-exams, when you walk your fingers in concentric circles around your breast and under your armpits. Practice self-exams lying down and standing up, and watch yourself in a mirror.

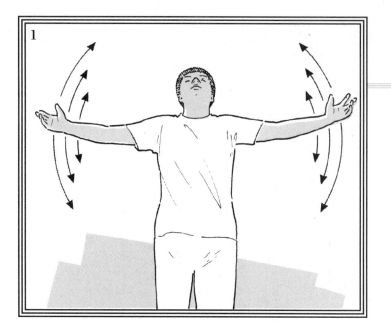

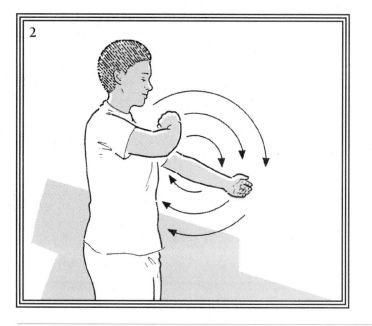

"Drawing Circles"—Breast Health and Postmastectomy Exercises

1. Breathe deeply. On the inhalation, raise and extend your arms slowly to the sides, exhale and lower them, inhale and raise them, like a bird flying in slow motion.
2. Raise your hands in front of you and draw slow circles, increasing the size of the circle each day.

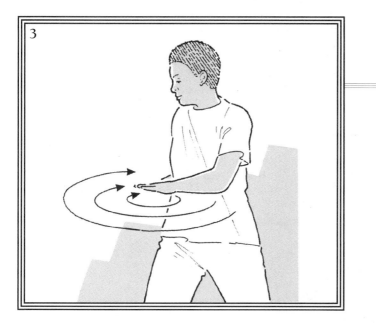

3. Start with your hands at your waist and extend them to the side to draw slow, horizontal circles.

4. Extend your arm in front of you and raise it slowly, increasing the lift each day until you can draw a vertical circle over your head. This will take the longest to achieve postmastectomy, so don't rush it.

In postmastectomy situations, practice a little each day until you can achieve complete circles. Practice to your favorite music, and hold a picture in your mind of yourself in glowing health.

PART II

PREVENTING INJURY

A. COMPUTER WORKERS

In the United States a class-action suit is pending against the major computer manufacturers on behalf of thousands of operators suffering from repetitive stress injuries. The most common problem is chronic carpal tunnel syndrome, when swollen tissues pinch the nerve running through the wrist, initially causing pins and needles in the fingers, then severe pain and, at worst, loss of muscle function. Manufacturers argue it's not the equipment, it's the way you use it.

Computer-damaged workers disagree, and many are willingly becoming involved in research on what the World Health Organization defines as "work related musculoskeletal disorders." Designers are testing split and tilted keyboards and simpler push-button systems to help alleviate the problems. But until something is done on a mass scale to improve the ergonomic design of keyboards and work areas, and workload, the problem will reach epidemic proportions. In Germany, by law, operators take a ten-minute break each hour from their computers. Similarly, the Japanese government limits the time workers spend at keyboards.

According to Jane E. Brody of the *New York Times* (March 3 and 4, 1992), computer-related hand and arm injuries account for up to 40 percent of workers' compensation claims in the United States. And newspaper reporters and editors worldwide are suffering from high rates of injury because of excessive work on computers.

Ophthalmologists in Europe and North America report increasing cases of computer-related eyestrain, and advise patients to glance away from the screen as often as they can and take proper breaks.

I became more sensitive to an assortment of computer-related health problems—and the devastating effects they can have on people's lives—after investing in a laptop computer. At first I couldn't understand why my eyes seemed to be pointing in all directions after a workday, why my neck and shoulders felt so stiff, why I got so irritable, or why, after intensive days, I felt out of touch, abstract, headachy, and sometimes nauseous.

Sound familiar?

These little electronic marvels have revolutionized our workday, but unless we adjust our work rhythm to alleviate the side effects, we're in for deep trouble. A high-pressure or deadline situation aggravates the problem.

Planning a little workday workout is not a big deal, especially if you're self-employed, but computer rooms are fast becoming today's equivalent of sweatshops.

There's little corporate recognition of the long-term consequences of work loss through recurring or chronic health problems, in contrast to the benefits—to all—of a workday with time built in for exercise and breaks. It may take multimillion-dollar lawsuits for the point to sink in.

There are various ways you can help prevent repetitive stress symptoms from building up. Maximize your work environment. Some people enjoy dolling up their computers with flowers and fun objects, like Whoopi Goldberg's terminal in the popular movie *Jumpin' Jack Flash*. But get the basics right first.

- Be conscious of your posture.
- Make sure your chair supports your back and your legs. Sit with comfortable right angles (back/upper legs, knees/floor). Your feet should be flat on the floor, with plenty of leg space. An adjustable swivel chair is best, ensuring support for the small of your back and easy mobility. An adjustable worktable is also advised.
- The screen should be set at eye level at a distance of some eighteen inches.
- The keyboard should be an extension of your hands.
- Angle your lamp away from you, so light bounces off the wall and won't create glare or reflections on the screen. Find a comfortable happy medium between a modified room light and sufficient light at your desk for you to see your screen and work documents.
- Use a viewer-friendly screen or add a screen cover.

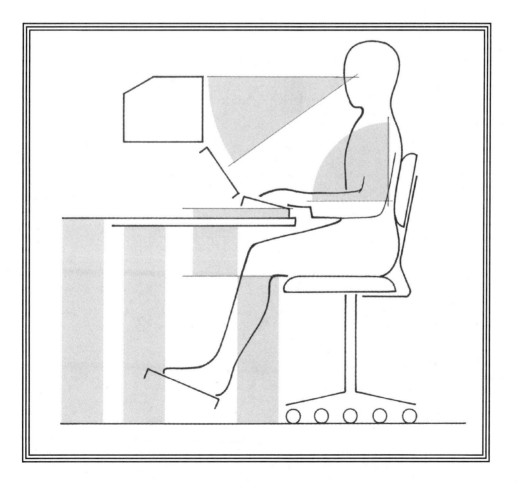

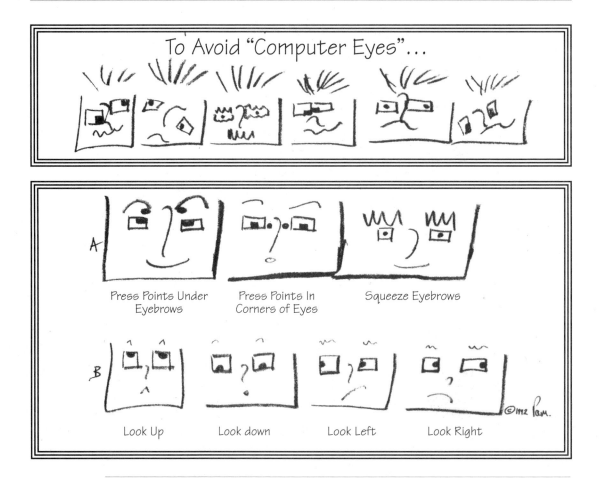

To Avoid "Computer Eyes"...

A — Press Points Under Eyebrows · Press Points In Corners of Eyes · Squeeze Eyebrows

B — Look Up · Look down · Look Left · Look Right

Daily Workout

- Stretch your arms and legs before you sit down.
- Do neck rolls. Look left. Look right. Squeeze down the back of your neck and across each shoulder.
- Tap imaginary lines stretching from your eyebrows, up your forehead, across the top of your head, and down your neck.
- Train yourself to look away from the computer screen every now and again. As a reminder, pin something on the wall facing you, something funny or colorful, anything to attract your eye away from the screen occasionally.
- To prevent wrist tension, rotate and flex your wrists before you start working.

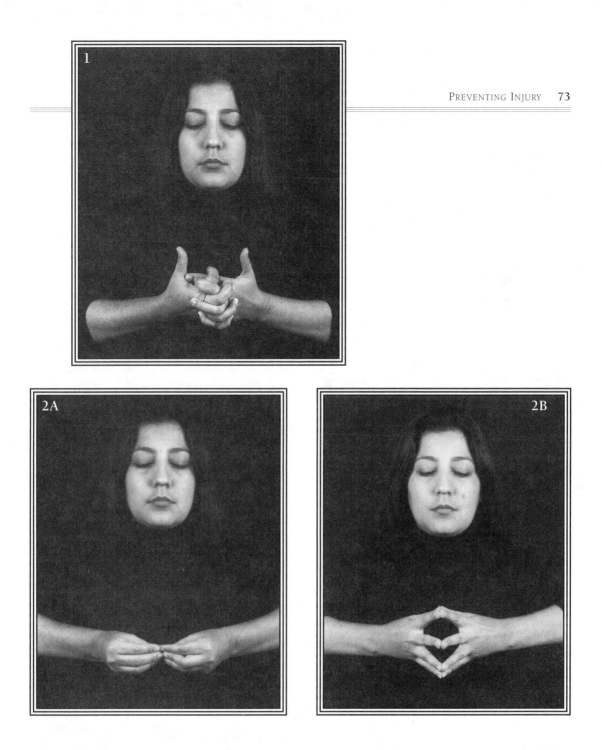

1. "Braid" your fingers. Move them back and forth.
2. Do "spider on the mirror" push-ups (**2A, 2B**).

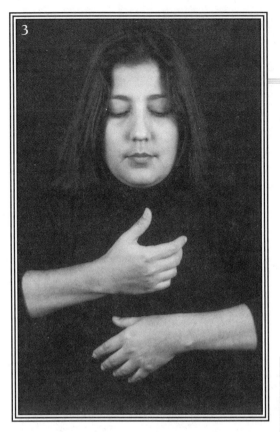

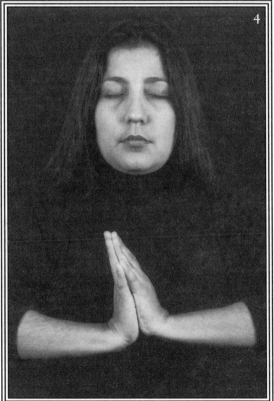

3. Do the "waterwheel." Hold hands in front of you, palms facing you. Now make rapid circles with your hands, one over the other, without touching.

4. Press your hands in the prayer position and move them from side to side.

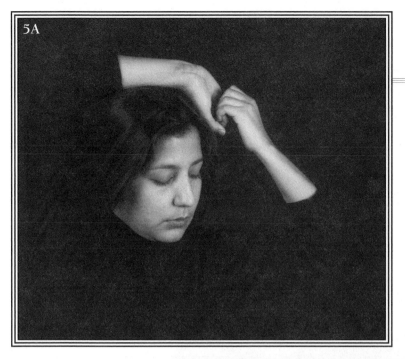

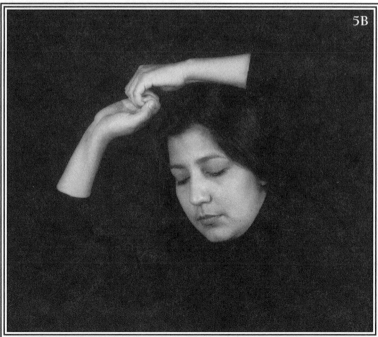

5 A, 5B. Grip your hands together behind your head and pull. Great for shoulder tension.

Mix 'n' match the exercises and repeat them at intervals during the day.

B. JOGGERS AND OTHER FITNESS FREAKS

I learned about the vulnerable points and lines of a jogger's body after years of running around New York's Central Park and hard streets in the sweltering humidity, razor-like winds, and driving rains. Neck, lower back, knees, shins, Achilles tendons, and feet all took a lot of punishment. Today it hurts me to see people pounding and puffing their way along the tarmac, believing they are doing wonders for their bodies.

For me, the harder the ground the better. It was faster. Chiropractors warned me about the impact on discs and suggested sand, grass, or soft ground, but being young and invincible, I needed my daily sweat and high, and thought extra stretching and yoga provided all the necessary cross-training. I went through a series of mini- and half-marathons in training for the New York Marathon until, one cold morning, I snapped a hamstring while demonstrating an exercise in a shiatsu class. I despaired. I'm ashamed to admit this, but I tried to run a day after the injury and fell to my knees. Countless runners have tried to jog through their injuries, which is why I mention it, so others can learn from such madness.

After receiving some deep-muscle repair work from chiropractor Dr. Dick Kowal, I bought a secondhand racing bike, joined a gym, did more brisk walking and swimming, and actually enjoyed the switch.

Some advice I've gathered along the way:

• Heed the warning signs and cross-train if you can. Mix 'n' match with cycling, walking, yoga, tai chi, weights, volleyball, anything. Don't wait for an injury to take you out. Run on softer ground as much as you can or switch to race walking.

• Don't neglect your stretching, before and after jogging. Warm up those tight muscles in cold weather. Walk before you jog.

• Coordinate your breathing with each step (inhale, 2, 3, 4, exhale, 2, 3, 4, or, when you speed up, inhale, 2, 3, exhale, 2, 3). You won't puff and pant like your fellow joggers. Your breath will fuel and not fight you. You'll be amazed at how calm you'll be.

• Integrate a few of the following self-shiatsu exercises with your stretching routine before and after your workout. In time you'll develop other "press and stretch" techniques. Take your time.

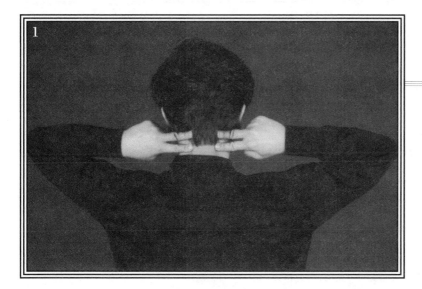

Daily Workout

Useful before and after jogging or any form of exercise.

1. "V" the index and middle fingers of both hands and press the back of your neck.
2. Roll your knuckles down either side of your spine.

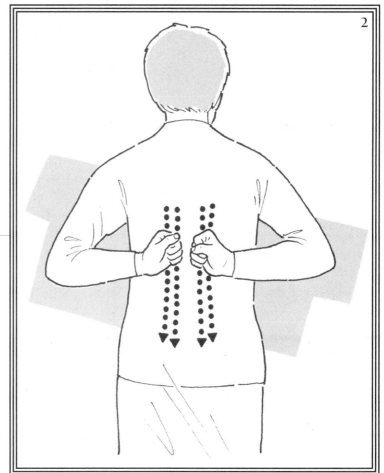

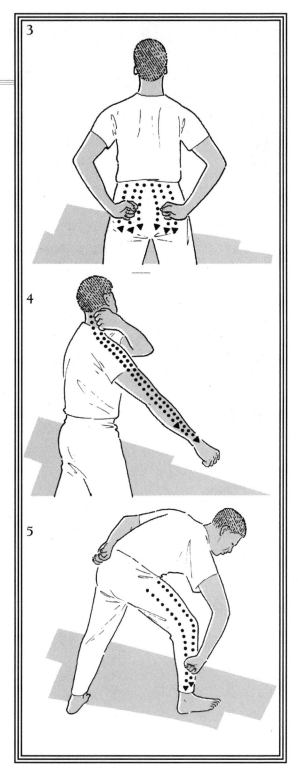

3. Work your knuckles around your butt and sacrum.
4. Work your knuckles down the side of your neck, across shoulders, and down your arms.
5. Work your knuckles down the sides of your legs.

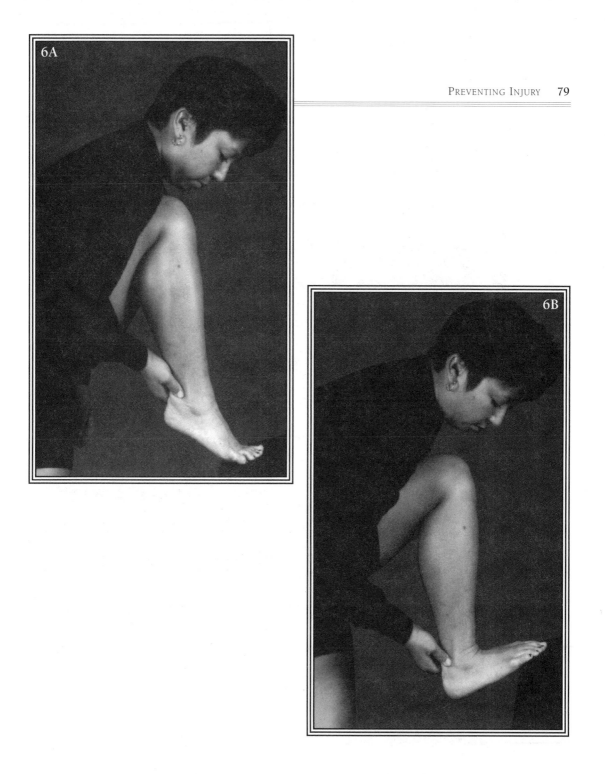

6A, 6B. Place foot on a stool. Pinch Achilles tendon while raising and lowering foot.

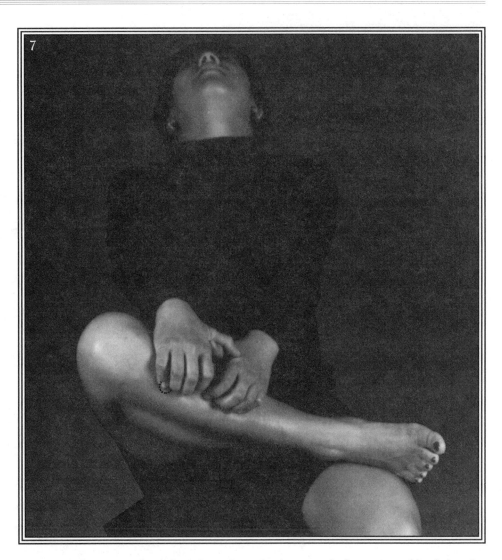

7. Sit, one leg crossed on the other. Grip shinbone with fingertips of both hands, lean back, and work down, arms straight. The first point you hit (see circle) may be especially sensitive. It's a key runner's point. In bygone days in the Orient, travelers would press this point after walking long distances, for energy, and to relieve tired legs. Jogging taught me why. This is the area that often hurts after you run some ten miles. Press it when you pause for water breaks. (We press this same area for menstrual pain. See section on menstruation.)

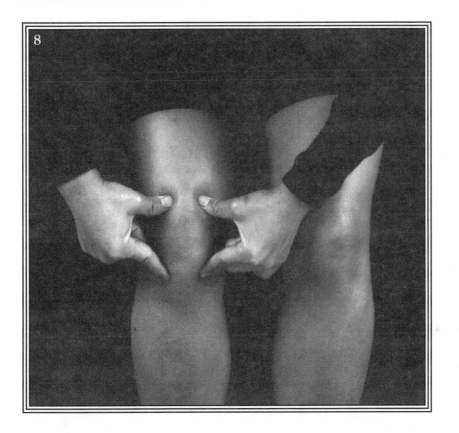

8. Press points above and below knees.

C. FREQUENT FLIERS

Crisscrossing the Atlantic as a child created the mosaic of my life. My work as a writer and teacher continues to involve a lot of transatlantic traveling. Perhaps it all started when my mother was pregnant with me. My parents and two small brothers experienced a nightmarish voyage from Cape Town to New York on the ill-fated liner *El Nil* during 1943 at the peak of the battle for the Atlantic in World War II. Then they traveled by train from New York to El Paso, Texas. As a child, I suffered from motion sickness when our lives continued to zigzag, from Mexico (where I was born) to various parts of North America, Europe, and Africa, because my father was a restless American geologist.

I soon learned that curling up like a pretzel made me nauseated, while slow breathing and sitting up straight helped to calm the queasiness. As an adult, especially while flying frequently between London and the Middle East, I took Dramamine to alleviate airsickness and an unpleasant sensation of walking about three feet off the ground for days after landing. During the mid-1970s in London my life moved into vegetarianism, meditation, and yoga, and I weaned myself off Dramamine. My instinctive deep breathing as a child mellowed into a practical way of utilizing intervals during flying, maybe ten minutes an hour, for meditation and relaxation.

Now, before entering a different time zone, I visualize the hands of the clock going forward or backward to landing time, and reset my watch before arrival so I step off the flight prepared.

By drinking a lot of bottled water (to counteract the dehydrating effects of flying) and requesting a vegetarian meal or fruit plate, I avoid that "weighed down" feeling. Ginger tea helps prevent nausea.

After my shiatsu training in the early 1980s, I began to experiment with in-flight exercises. Practicing them for five or ten minutes each hour has proved to be a wonderful way of traveling comfortably. Fellow passengers often ask me to teach them.

In 1992 I was delighted to discover British Airways offered booklets of similar exercises for passengers, and a meditation channel along with jazz and classical music.

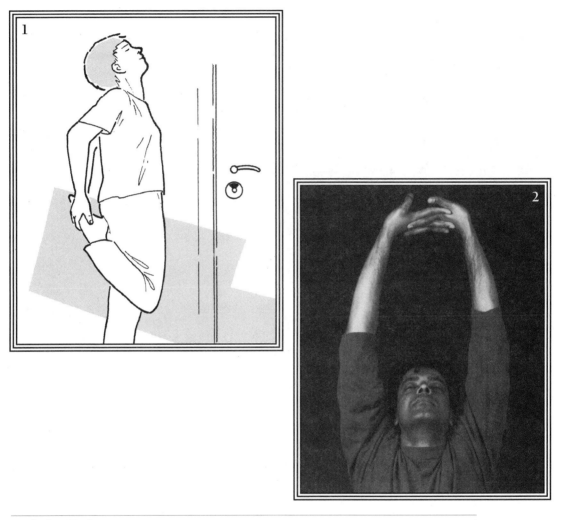

In-flight Workout

1. Utilize those moments when you are waiting in line for the toilet to stretch your legs by bending one knee at a time, reaching back, and grabbing hold of your foot.
2. When you feel cramped, uncomfortable, or claustrophobic while flying, remember the space above your head. Stretch and look up. You'll be amazed at the effect.

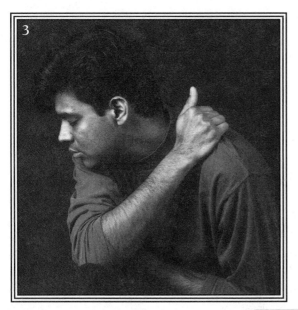

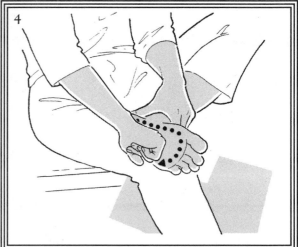

3. When you start to feel restless in your seat, rotate your head. Look left. Look right. Squeeze across your shoulders.

4. Raise your left foot on your right knee. Remove your shoe. Make a fist and work around the sole of your foot in a clockwise direction. Then do the right foot. Wiggle your toes and rotate your ankles.

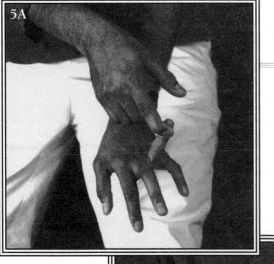

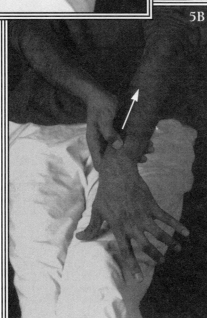

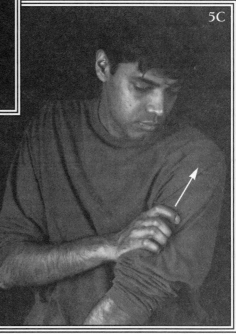

5. With your palm facing down, lift your ring
   finger with your other hand (**5A**). Imagine
   a line that runs from your ring finger up
   along the middle of your arm to your
   shoulder (**5B, 5C**). Don't be in a hurry. Pressure should be firm and slow. Then do the
   other arm. (You are stimulating the meridian
   that helps you adapt to change and boosts
   the immune system.)

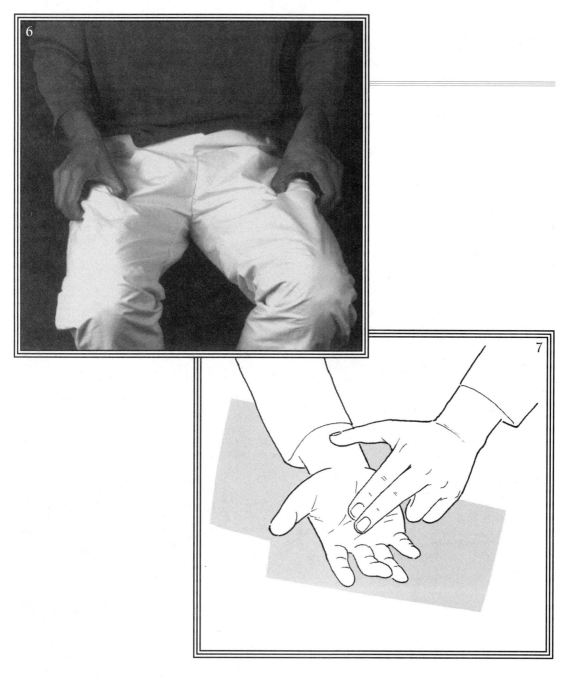

6. Pinch down the tops of your legs toward your knees. Flex your knees. Then continue down, pinching your shinbone to your ankles. Great way to relieve cramped legs.

7. If you feel afraid, simply place one hand on your knee, palm up. Rest the fingers of your other hand on your palm, your thumb just below your wrist.

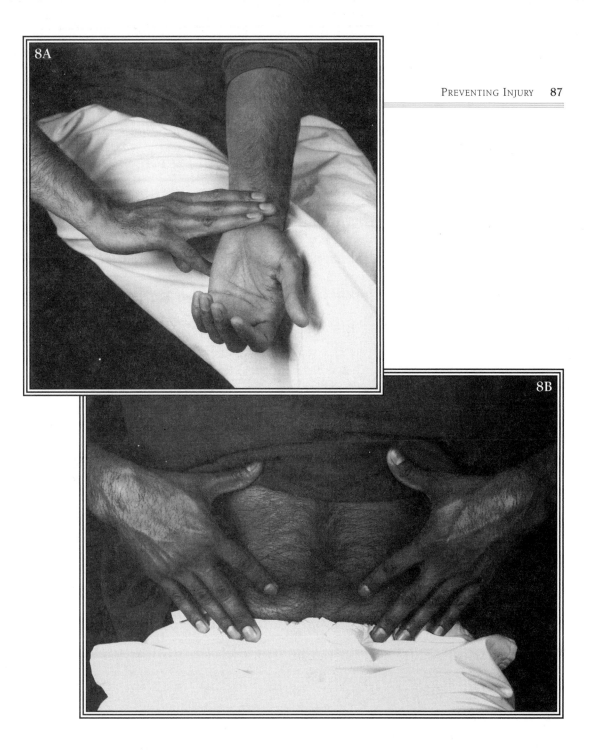

8. If you feel nauseated, apply pressure to the point just three finger widths from your wrist **(8A)**. Also press points about one inch on either side of your navel **(8B)**.

To complement your in-flight workout:

- Repeat all of the above (or some of it) each hour. You'll step off the flight refreshed and exercised.
- Try to exercise when you reach your destination. A brisk walk will do wonders. So will swimming, but if this isn't practical, then spend half an hour stretching. If your flight is delayed or you're holed up at an airport for hours in transit, walk around briskly or stretch beside your seat. People won't think you're crazy. They often join in and stretch with you!
- When you arrive, expose yourself to light or sunlight as much as possible. This helps to reset your biological clock. Stop saying to yourself, "Oh, it's 2 A.M. in New York, or 9 P.M. in London," when your body is busily adapting to local time. Flights from the U.S. to Europe are frequently overnight, so after you've exercised, go through the breakfast ritual (even if you just nibble half a croissant and drink something hot) to get you into the rhythm of the new time zone. Similarly, when you return to the U.S. from Europe in midafternoon, exercise to stay awake as long as you can, eat something light (a small salad) at suppertime, and you'll probably sleep the night through.
- Continue to drink bottled water and eat whole foods, fresh fruit, and veggies. Natural yogurt is a great way of helping your intestines to harmonize with local foods. A young Greek doctor on the island of Skyros told me this many years ago, and it always works.
- Avoid flopping down in a hotel room trying to unwind in front of a TV. This confuses your biological clock and you'll spend days trying to adjust to local time or culture shock.

Try all or at least some of the above exercises, and see what a difference they make to your next traveling experience.

PART III

SPREADING GOOD HEALTH

FAMILY SHIATSU

It's a joy when students try out some of the techniques of our workshops on their own families, their partners, kids, and elderly relatives. As receivers and givers, children are especially responsive to shiatsu and related stretching techniques. You can also try some of the techniques on your animals. One of my former students in Switzerland, Christine Urben, found shiatsu and rotation techniques to be the only method that helped ease pain and stiffness in the hip of her Bernese mountain dog. Others have used shiatsu to ease stressed muscles in their horses and as health maintenance for cats and guinea pigs.

In family terms, even just the simplest forms of stretching and pressure point work tune you into the essence of shiatsu as folk healing and prevention against illness. You can also make good use of some basic techniques if you are taking care of a sick or disabled relative at home.

Feel free to experiment. Use the following exercises as a rough guideline, and enjoy the new techniques that often evolve quite spontaneously.

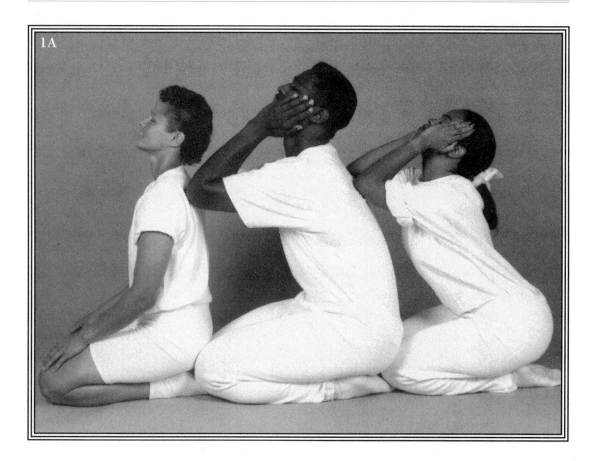

1A

A. FAMILY EXERCISES

Here are some warm-up techniques:

1A. Whether you work with your partner, your child, or as a family group, you can have a lot of fun sitting elbows-to-back (lined up like a train). You'll discover some lovely variations, like feet-to-shoulders (**1B**), and then "walking" down backs with your feet or your knuckles (**1C**). Remember—no pressure on the spine.

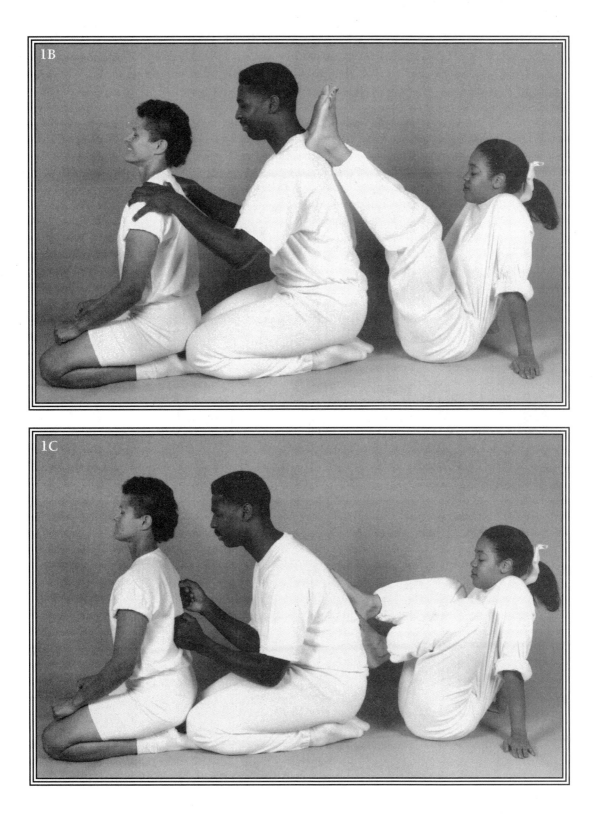

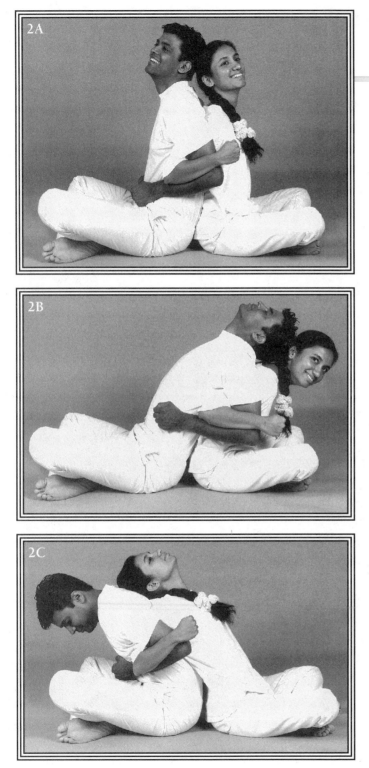

2A–C. When you sit back-to-back, make sure you are as close together as possible. Legs can be straight or crossed, whatever feels more comfortable. Link arms. Lean forward and back, forward and back, slowly and evenly. You'll feel a good, arched stretch. Super way to ease back and shoulder tension.

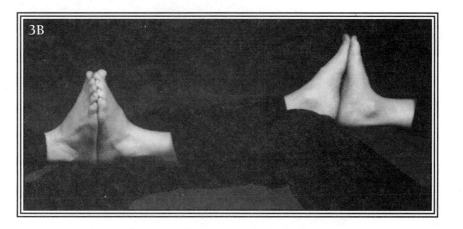

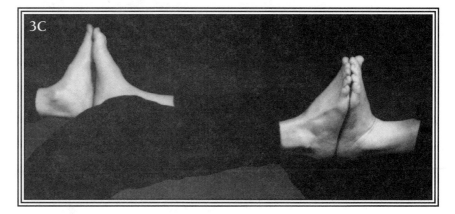

3A–C. *Feet-to-feet.* Lie on your backs with your legs raised, feet pointed and
   pressed together. Lie far enough apart so you can move your legs back and
   forth, back and forth, together, alternately, and in a circle, like a bicycle. Great
   for releasing back, shoulder, and leg stiffness. Once you've got the rhythm
   going, your legs will create all kinds of patterns.

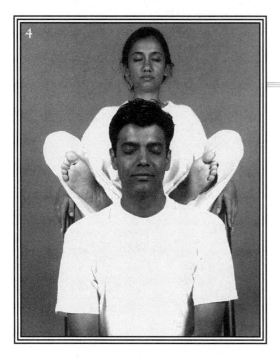

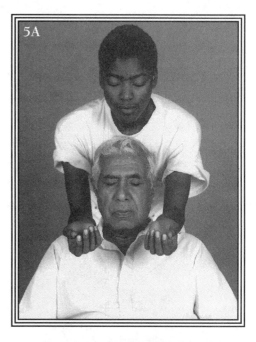

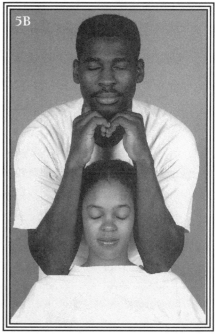

4. *Feet-to-Shoulders.* Sit on a chair and ask your partner to sit on the floor. Rest your feet or heels on your partner's shoulders. Great for shoulder tension.

5. You can also try resting your forearms (**5A**) or elbows (**5B**) on your partner's tight shoulders.

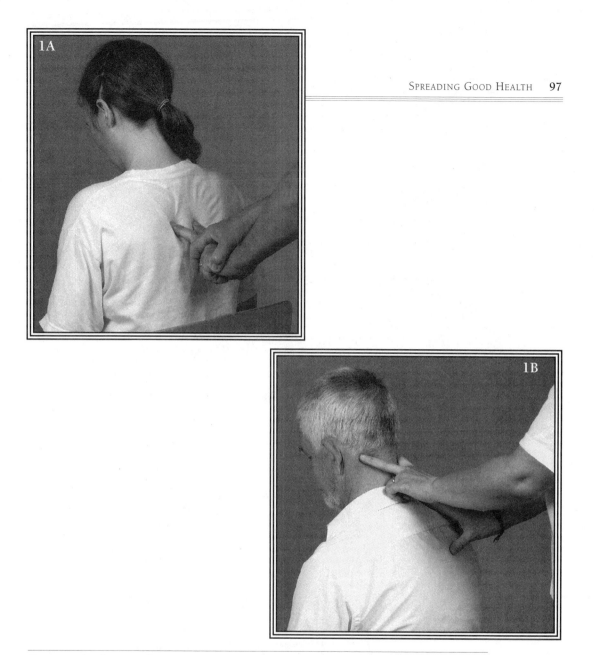

Once you've loosened up, you can start experimenting with the following:

1. Make a V of your first and second fingers and stroke down either side of your partner's spine (**1A**). Then imagine a row of dots down either side of the spine. Use your V or two thumbs to press two dots simultaneously. Never put any pressure on the spine itself. "V" down the back when the person is sitting, lying, or in baby pose. "V" along occipital ridge for headaches (**1B**).

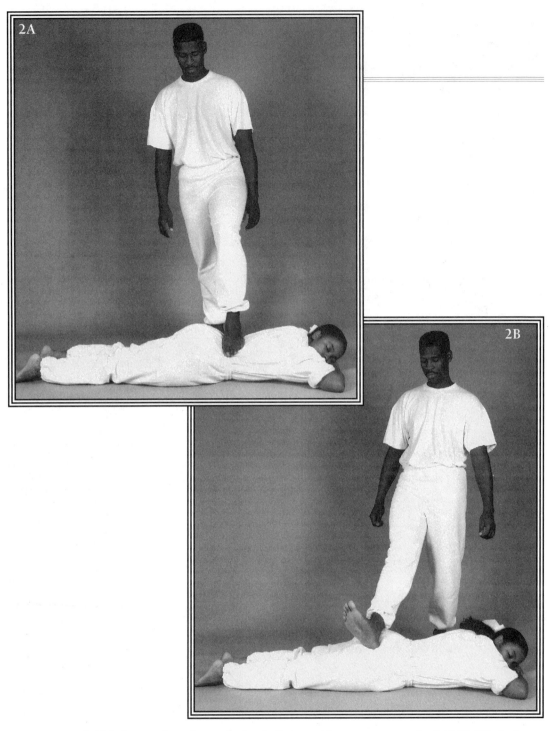

2. Work your foot down the back (but avoid pressure on spine) (**2A**). Work down butt (**2B**), and legs (**2C**). Rest elbows on butt in baby pose (**2D**).

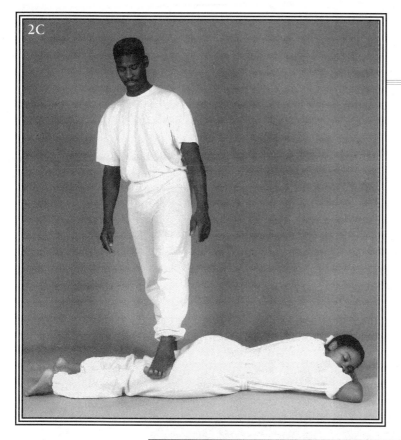

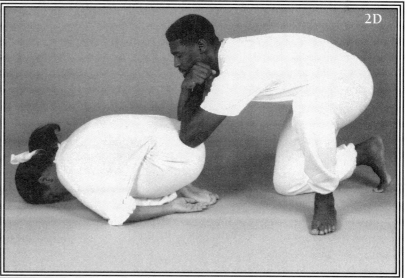

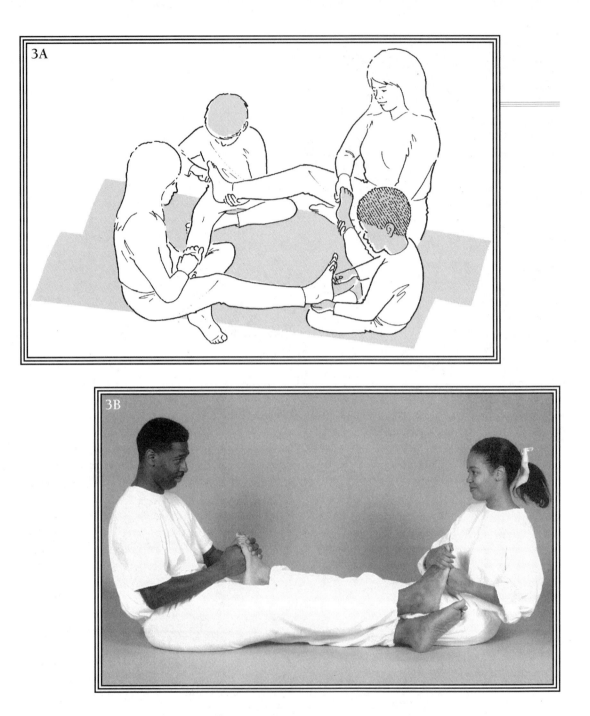

3. Sit in a circle. Place your right foot on the thigh of the person seated on your right, so each of you is holding a right foot (**3A**). Adjust positions so all of you are comfy. Give and receive simultaneously. Or just two of you can sit opposite one another (**3B**).

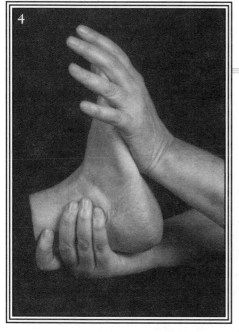

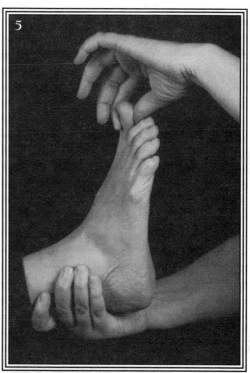

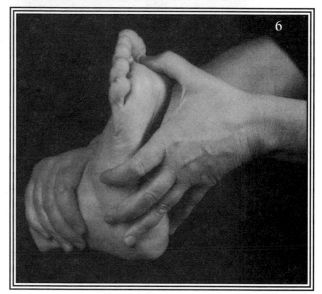

4. Hold the foot with one hand
and rotate it with the other.

5. Pull each toe in turn.

6. Press the base of each toe.

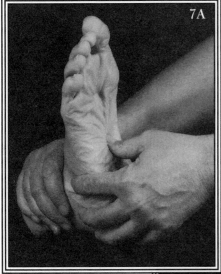

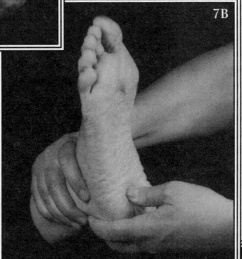

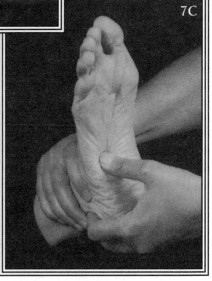

7A–C. Thumb or knuckle your way around sole of foot in a clockwise direction.

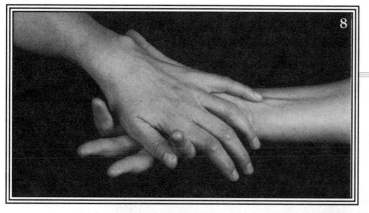

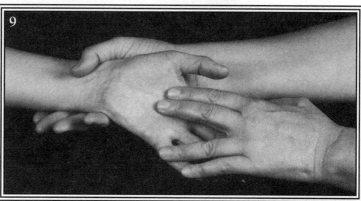

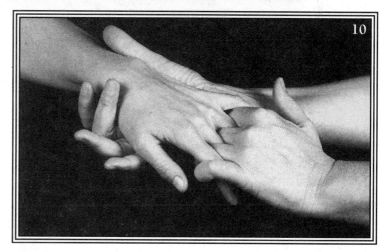

Now work on one another's hands.

8. If you need to calm someone, let palm rest on palm.
9. Then gently rest fingers on palm, and thumb on wrist.
10. Interlace fingers, squeeze, and pull. Then pull each finger.

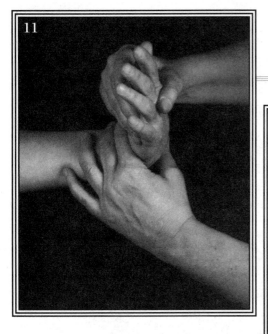

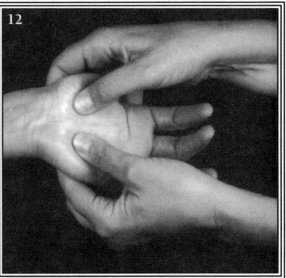

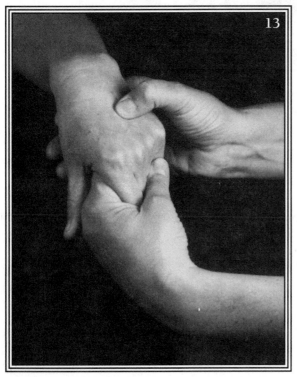

11. Flex and rotate wrist, slowly and evenly.
12. Press thumbs around palm.
13. Work down between metacarpals.

In the case of a sick spouse or child, work a lot on hands and feet, but slowly, evenly, and gently.

Practice hand and foot work in your family as often as you can. It is one of the most beautiful shiatsu gifts to receive, and to teach, and has been used for generations across many different cultures as a classic form of prevention against disease. The whole body benefits. If you practice hand and foot work each week, you'll feel very comfortable with the technique when you nurse a sick spouse, child, or friend, visit someone in the hospital, or help a loved one through the process of dying.

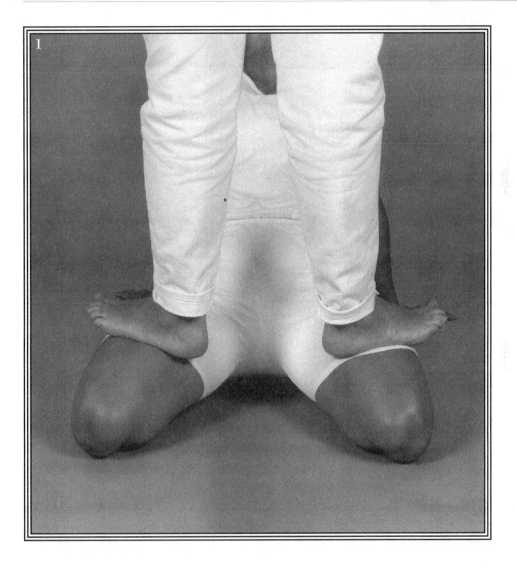

Exercises for Menstrual Pain to Do with a Friend

1. Kneel on the floor and lean back on your hands. Partner rests hands on your shoulders and walks up your thighs, feet out like Charlie Chaplin. Avoid this exercise if you have knee problems.

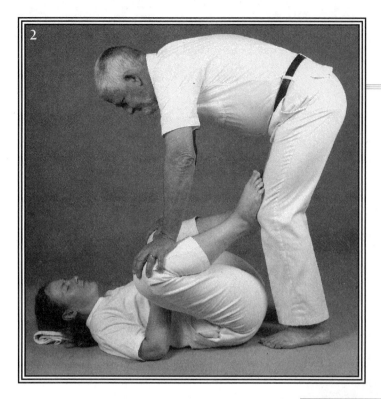

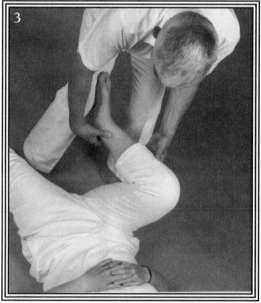

2. Press your knees to your chest.
3. Partner presses points below knee (outside shin bone), and four fingers width up from ankle on inside leg, simultaneously. (See section on self-shiatsu for menstruation.)

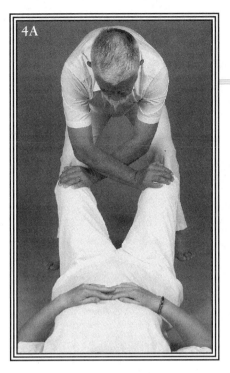

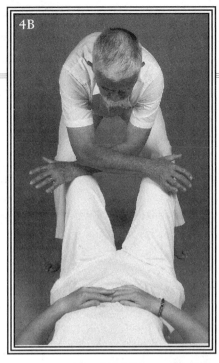

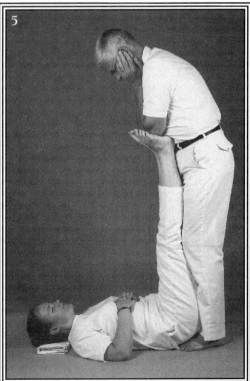

4. Partner presses the inside of your knees with crossed hands as you exert counter-pressure (**4A**). Partner releases hands suddenly (**4B**). Often a swift way of ending a cramp.

5. Partner supports your raised legs, and leans elbows on your feet. Super for menstrual and lower back pain.

B . Pregnancy, Labor, and Delivery

Regular shiatsu is a wonderful way of relaxing and easing back pain, weary legs, constipation, or morning sickness during pregnancy. It is also great during a long labor and in the delivery room. I have helped many women through pregnancy and delivery, and learn something new from each and every one to share in my classes— especially with midwives.

If you are unable to receive professional shiatsu, you and your husband, partner, or a friend can benefit from a few simple techniques to make this an enrichingly shared experience. Practice a lot during the months of pregnancy, so you will find it easier to apply the techniques during labor and delivery.

Of course regular exercise is of paramount importance, and swimming will be most beneficial in the final months. One of my Swiss students, midwife Annemarie Kalasek of Frauenfeld, invited fellow teacher Erika Bringold and me to join one of her classes with pregnant women in the pool at the Universitatsspital (Zürich's teaching hospital). She gave the women back shiatsu underwater. When they floated face-up, she supported them under the sacrum with her knuckles to ease lower back pain.

She held their hands and pulled them around in slow, graceful circles, then had them develop breathing techniques. The group experience was not only instructional but a lot of fun.

If you smoke or drink, make a supreme effort to quit during pregnancy and create a smoke-free home—you owe it to yourself and your unborn child. If you start to crave certain foods (often sweet or salty foods), see if your body is signaling some vitamin or mineral deficiency, and make sure you are replacing it efficiently with supplements advised by your physician. If you experience morning sickness, try tapping your breastbone. Try eating sugarless oatmeal cookies or salt-free soda crackers.

Some women exercise a lot up until the final days—yoga, cycling, swimming, tai chi, or whatever. Exercises that stretch and open the inner thighs are especially important.

Women who are restricted for one reason or another during the final weeks can utilize the hands and feet "pebble therapy" (p. 45) to keep energy stimulated.

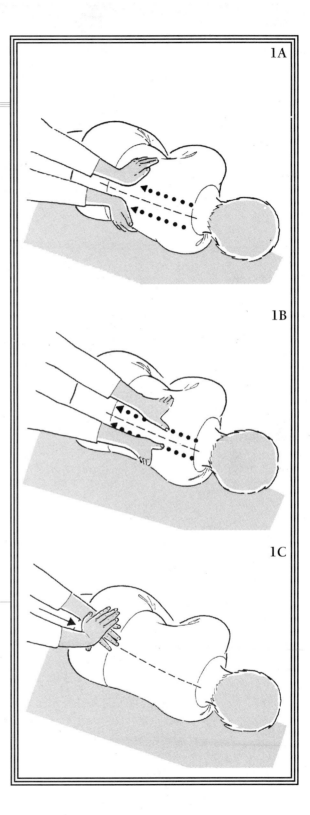

Shiatsu for the Pregnant Woman

1. Work down her back in the side
   position, by pressing your hands
   (**1A**) and then your thumbs (**1B**)
   down either side of her spine. Place
   your hands (or feet) flat on her
   sacrum (**1C**). The latter is a very
   releasing technique for lower back
   pain.

2. To ease weary or painful legs, especially at the end of the day, place your hands on either side of her ankle and slide them up to her thighs and around under her hips. Repeat on the other side.

3. Work feet and hands as much as you can. (See section on family exercises.)

4. Place your hands gently on her abdomen. Move hands in slow, clockwise circles. Right hand leads, and passes under left hand. Very soothing and connecting for all three of you!

Shiatsu During Labor

1. Continue using the back techniques you've perfected during the last few months. Palm or thumb your way down her back on either side of the spine, during, after, and between contractions. This may last from four to forty-eight hours!

   Depending on what sort of breathing technique she is using (deep breathing or the Lamaze "panting" technique), she will soon tell you if she prefers you to work down her back during a contraction, or just support her upper, mid, or lower back or sacrum with both your hands. If she is lying on her side on the floor, or in bed, you can save your hands from becoming tired or stiff by using your feet or your elbows, especially on her sacrum.

2. Work on her feet and lower back a lot between contractions.

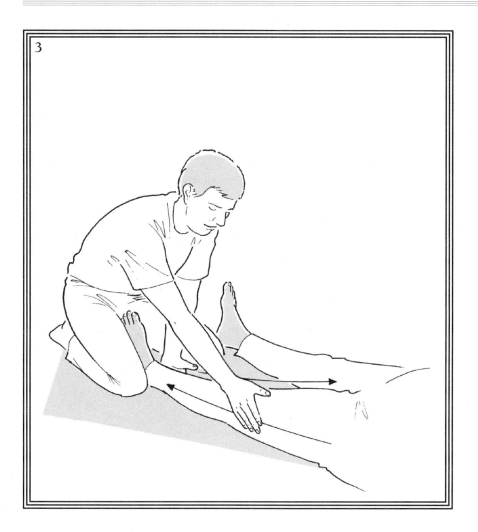

3. To keep energy moving in her legs, place one hand inside her ankle and the other hand outside her knee, and "sweep" your hands toward one another (always up on the inside and down on the outside). Practice this a few times to achieve a smooth coordination, and repeat on the other side.

4. If she can experience most of her labor at home, she will move around, squat, hang off you, crawl, and find countless different body positions for comfort, or to ease pain. Just move around with her. She may also find it helpful to sit on a stool (and lean on a table) while you squeeze her buttocks.

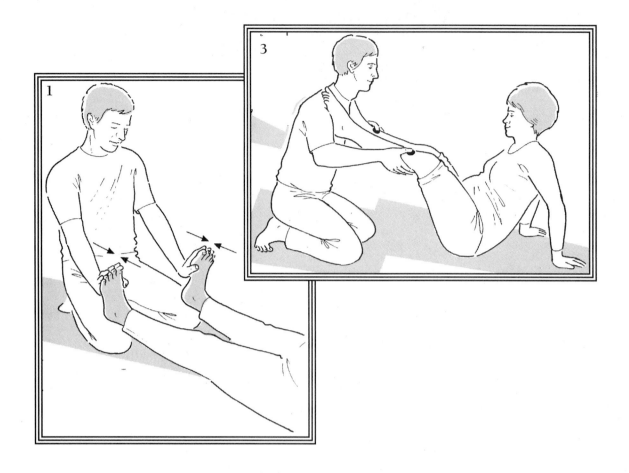

Shiatsu During Delivery

1. When the physician, nurse, or midwife says she has dilated sufficiently and can start pushing during contractions, you can help by applying counterpressure against her feet with your hands or knuckles.

2. Press the points we use for menstruation (just below the knee on the outside of the leg, and four fingers up from the ankle on the inside). Also press her little toe (especially the outer corner of the nail) as hard as you can.

3. In the final hour (or hours) when she starts her massive pushing in the delivery room, press these points fiercely. If attending doctors or midwives can't work around a squat delivery, the most natural childbirth posture, and she must sit with her legs raised, then access the leg points when she pushes her feet against your chest or shoulders (or she can push one leg against you and one against someone on the other side of the bed).

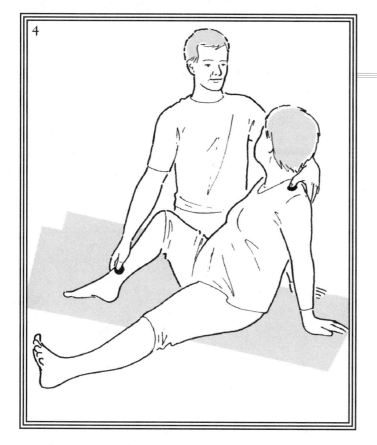

4. Adjust your position to press one point on her shoulder and the point above the ankle, simultaneously. Or you can sit behind her and support her.

5. If her hemorrhoids bother her and prevent her from pushing, you can numb the pain by holding an ice pack under her anus.

6. Between the actual "crowning" (when you can see the top of the baby's head) and the baby's entrance, push the leg points as hard as you can as she pushes, and ease up as she inhales, so your rhythm matches hers.

Don't be afraid to stop and start the point-pushing techniques in between procedures, such as an epidural (a shot to numb the lower extremities) or an episiotomy (incision into the perineum and vagina to prevent tearing during delivery).

Shiatsu After Delivery

- Continue pressing points on legs and feet until the placenta is expelled. Shiatsu can help speed up this process.
- To help uterine tone an hour or two after delivery, squeeze the tops of her legs from thigh down to ankle.

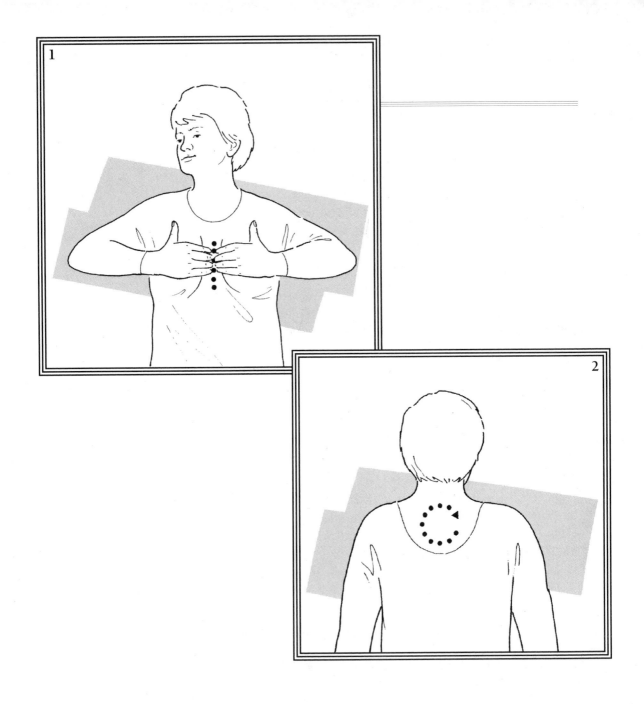

Breast Feeding

1. If she is having problems while she is breast-feeding, encourage her to press points between her breasts.

2. Work around a circle at the top of her back.

After Delivery

Depending on the nature of the delivery and her energy level, our new mama may want to sleep around the clock, or she may appreciate some shiatsu on her back, legs, feet, and hands.

After I helped one young single parent give birth to her first baby, she asked, "Who mothers the mother?"

This is a time for a lot of nurturing, to replenish energy and to combat postpartum blues. Fathers, especially those deeply involved in the pregnancy and delivery, also need a lot of nurturing. Some 50 percent of husbands or partners of women experiencing postpartum depression suffer from a similar depression, according to studies done by Dr. Simon Lovestone of the Maudsley Institute of Psychiatry in London (*The Independent on Sunday*, March 29, 1994).

Fears of sudden parenthood and future responsibilities can put a dark spin on moods and behavior following childbirth, and many marital problems can stem from this time if the situation isn't recognized and dealt with. But the subject is still something of a taboo because it contradicts the joyful image of birth.

Many couples are helped by turning to ancient rituals for celebrating the placenta, instead of allowing it to be whisked away for disposal—or sent to pharmaceutical companies to be used in a variety of medications (a practice recently banned in Britain). Different customs, different rituals. Some Native American tribes bury it in the mountains or under a tree, which is then revered by the child. In some areas of South Africa the placenta is buried under the front door of the house, and in some parts of West Africa divining is done from the placenta, or it is formally buried as the baby's "twin."

Stillbirth, Miscarriage, or Abortion

Gentle shiatsu (especially for the back and feet) can be very healing and soothing in cases of stillbirth, miscarriage, and abortion.

Again, many couples turn to meditations or ancient rituals linked to their particular ancestry to help them cope with loss. The absence of rituals leaves a gap, a sense of unresolve, an anguish, and a subconscious search that can last for years.

Dennis Tresise, a monumental mason who has carved and chiseled generations of gravestones in his hometown of Redruth, Cornwall, told me that women come to him forty or fifty years after a stillbirth to find out if he knows where local hospitals buried their offspring in the days when that was the custom.

Rituals, even the simple scattering of flowers close to a place associated with either the loss or the conception, help to anchor emotional turmoil, grief, and help-lessness, in some sort of structure or framework. Medicine woman Shamaan Ochaum guides couples through such healing ceremonies for a sense of completion. She talks in cosmic terms about birth as a cocreation contract between parents and unborn child. For one reason or another, if the time isn't right for that child to be born, parents can honor this decision as a way of letting go.

A burial ceremony for the stillborn child or miscarried fetus helps ease the blunt loss. A similar ritual can help women who suffer needless guilt and pain after abor-tions. If it's not possible to bury the fetus, Ochaum encourages parents to bury something from their own bodies, a nail or a lock of hair, as a symbolic way of returning a similar substance to the universe.

C. Working With Your Children and Shiatsu

Children are naturals for shiatsu. They respond to the techniques quickly and easily, since they're in tune with their bodies in a way we often need to relearn as adults. Picasso said he took a lifetime to learn how to draw as a child does. The same could be said of shiatsu.

Group stretching and foot work are great ways of absorbing kids' energies on a rainy day, teaching them healthy skills for their entire lives. Try to perform a series of exercises in different positions so young kids don't get restless or bored. Creating names for the different exercises can make them special to your family as well.

My students who are parents tell me that simple ways of working on the back, feet, and hands can help their kids through sleeping problems, fear, sadness, bed-wetting, stomach pains, or hyperactivity. Others have helped kids through asthma attacks.

Start working on your kids at an early age, as a loving way of giving them preventive care. Kids are great imitators, so it won't be long before they want to work on *you*! I've also seen kids go off and practice on their dolls.

Again, as with all these exercises, use your common sense. A sudden or severe cramp, earache, or back pain needs to be checked immediately by a physician.

In my classes, children are often very clear about describing pain. During a workshop in New York, I remember talking to an eight-year-old boy who suffered from chronic headaches. His parents had taken him through the standard route of medical and eye examinations, and no physical cause could be found, so they were exploring other routes.

I asked him to show me where he experienced the pain. He touched points on his forehead, head, and neck. "Show me on the acupuncture chart," I suggested, handing him a box of colored pins.

"Wow, this is exactly where I feel the pain," he said, stabbing points associated with classic forms of headaches.

He showed me where the pain started and where it intensified. "Try pressing those points next time you feel a headache is on its way," I told him.

Some weeks later, he sent word to say the technique helped. No, the headaches hadn't stopped, but the pain was less intense and he felt he could control it.

The key here, of course, was involving the boy in his own healing process, and in a way that fired his imagination. I hear similar stories from pediatric nurses about the effectiveness of involving young patients in monitoring temperature readings, blood pressure, and so on, as a way of easing fear and pain and respecting the child's intelligence. No one pretends this is an instant cure, but it helps, and can also be a useful tip for parents who are nursing their kids back to health at home.

Dr. Elisabeth Kübler-Ross, world-renowned Swiss thanatologist, has done some extraordinary work with terminally ill children, their drawings, insights, and observations, all of which teach us to listen to a sick child and never underestimate his or her grasp of the situation. Drawings and paintings are especially revealing.

I remember an exhibition of hospitalized children's art in New York some years ago displayed in the windows of ABC-TV. Health professionals could have learned a lot. One picture showed a peanut-sized kid dwarfed by instruments and huge figures in white coats. Another showed a sad face over the caption "In the morning they go to the kitchen to 'unfresh' the bread."

Many children suffer pain needlessly in hospitals because, sadly, the subject has not been considered a top priority, according to reports in the nursing journal *Nurseweek* ("Children's Pain," Part 1, January 24, 1994; Part 2, February 1, 1994). In the current flurry of research to help a pediatric unit recognize pain signals often misunderstood in the past, much is being made of scales to evaluate pain through body language and facial and vocal expressions, especially in preverbal kids. Preschool kids are asked to point at one of a series of faces ranging from happy to gloomy to tearful or are given games involving crayons or poker chips.

Many parents will read this and say they know how to recognize pain in their own kids; why don't the nurses and doctors ask them? Clearly, two-way communication is vital.

There are many ways a loving parent can help alleviate pain in a hospitalized child, and the worst thing is for a parent to convey fear to a kid.

A friend stopped me in a street near Zürich some years ago, distraught. His eight-year-old son was hospitalized with burns from a gasoline explosion in a farmer's shed.

My friend felt helpless. He enjoyed a wonderful rapport with his son and believed in a lot of hugging and touching. But, because of the injuries, he wasn't able to hold and comfort his son.

"What about his feet?" I asked.

"His feet?"

"Sure. Were they burned?"

He shook his head.

I gave him books on shiatsu and reflexology, showed him how he could help ease his son's pain and discomfort and touch him in a way that was full of love and healing at the same time. Later he told me how much this simple exercise meant to them both, and how the boy soon told him which points helped to ease his pain.

These stories demonstrate very different situations where shiatsu offered an alternative approach to children and their problems. I stress, no "instant cure" was sought or given, but in each case I was struck by the openness of the kids.

Shiatsu students who are also parents love to share their own experiences. One Swiss student told me he worked regularly on his two-year-old daughter by telling her, "We'll plant some strawberries here and some raspberries here," as he pressed points along her arms. Each day she would look to see if the "berries" had started to sprout.

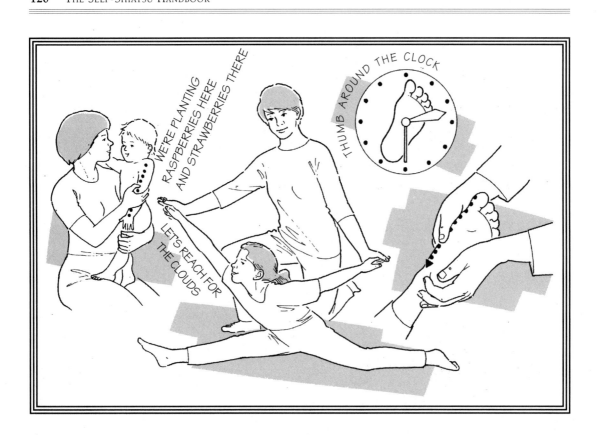

Some general advice when working with young children:

1. Depending on the age (and/or problem) of the child, make good use of stretching and imagery ("Let's pretend we're stretching like chewing gum, or E.T.'s finger," "Let's reach for the clouds," etc.).
2. Similarly, utilize the game "This little piggy went to market" to work on a child's toes. Work around soles with your thumb as though around the face of a clock ("Here's three o'clock, here's three-thirty . . ."). To calm hyperactivity, thumb your way along instep from big toe to heel.
3. Utilize different positions (sitting, side) with imagery, if the child gets restless.

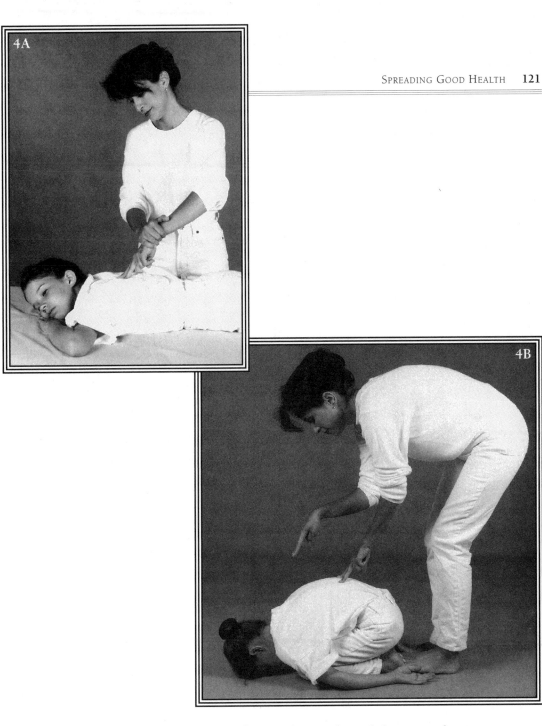

4. Make a V out of your first and second fingers. First stroke and then press down either side of the spine to help relax a child who is distressed, in pain, unable to sleep, or hyperactive (**4A**). "V" your way down child's back in baby pose (**4B**).

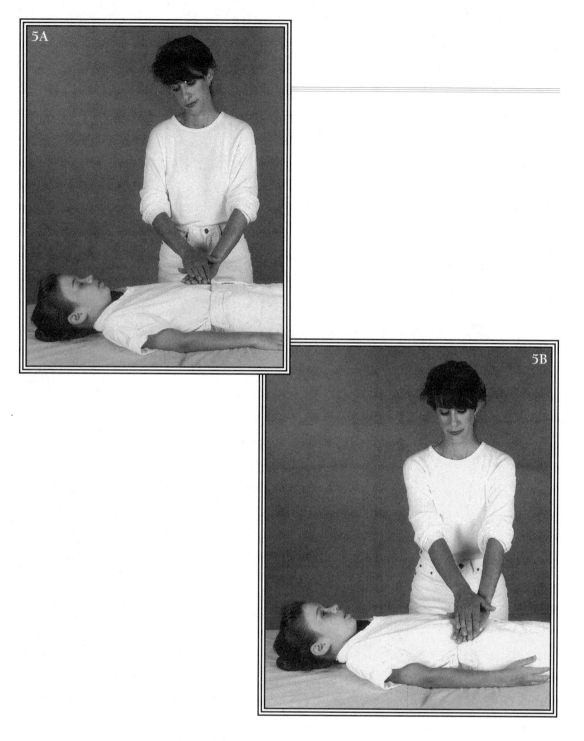

5A, 5B. To soothe a child, or to ease a stomachache, draw slow circles with the flat of your hand on his or her abdomen in a clockwise direction.

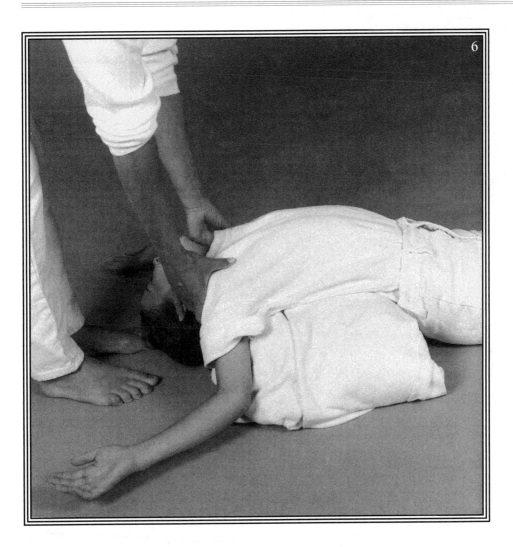

6. To help an asthmatic child, have your child lie on the floor faceup, back arched, resting on a cushion or your feet. Press underneath the collarbone to the shoulder. This position (simulating the fish pose of yoga) is also very good for back pain. Or stand behind your child, with your hands under his or her armpits.

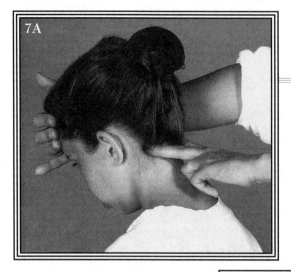

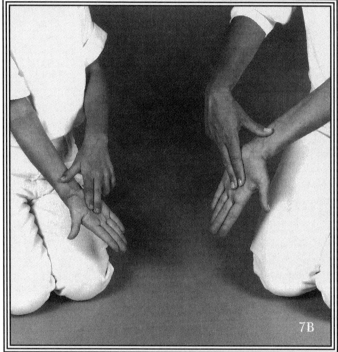

7. To help your children overcome travel sickness, make sure they sit up straight. Try pressing points under the occipital ridge, midway between ears and cervical vertebrae (**7A**). Rest your fingers on their palm and wrist, and encourage them to do this for themselves (**7B**).

In time, you and your kids will discover all kinds of variations for yourselves and have a lot of fun along the way.

D. SHIATSU FOR SENIOR CITIZENS

It's wonderful to see seventy- and eighty-year-old men and women doing yoga or tai chi, cycling or climbing mountains, and generally breaking all the silly stereotypes about aging. Of some 54 million senior Americans, about one-quarter work full-time and many more would like to work beyond retirement age. An estimated 1 million seniors are raising their grandchildren. As life expectancy rises (more for women than for men), the U.S. Census Bureau predicts the over-65s will reach 70 million, or 20 percent of the population, by 2030.

According to an article in the *New England Journal of Medicine* of January 28, 1993 (328:246–52), senior citizens are significant users of alternative medical therapies, a fact little known a few years ago in the United States. This means that shiatsu, with some encouragement, can look forward to even more growth in this sector of the population.

Peak fitness is not a prerequisite for shiatsu. Family exercises can be enjoyed by men and women who are still young at heart but perhaps not quite as agile as they once were. Couples of all ages can enjoy shiatsu exercises, and it's never too early—or too late—to start.

Grandparents and great-grandparents can benefit from the exercises, working together or with their kids or grandkids, or alone.

In older, more traditional societies, senior citizens are sought and revered for their wisdom, and often rule the household. In the West we've lost much of this. In the U.S., "Granny dumping" (abandoning senile relatives hundreds of miles from home) has become a sad symbol of the 1990s, and decent basic care for senior citizens is a luxury few can afford. We're all living longer and requiring more specialized forms of care in our dotage.

E. SHIATSU FOR SPECIAL CARE

Some Canadian nursing schools include classes such as Touch for Health in the curriculum and emphasize the needs of senior citizens.

Elisabeth Reichel, M.D., of Montreal points out the value of touch in geriatrics and used shiatsu in her former clinical practice and hospital rounds. She invited me to spend time with Alzheimer patients in a Montreal hospital, because she had discovered their responsiveness to touch and wanted me to teach the nurses a few shiatsu techniques.

I was struck by the way men and women suffering from Alzheimer paced up and down anxiously, often following patterns in the floor or lines around a wall.

The high level of anxiety and pacing made me modify shiatsu techniques to a few moments here and there. Working on shoulders, hands, legs, and feet proved most calming. But stress symptoms seemed far less exaggerated on wards where Alzheimer patients were not isolated as a group, but included with patients suffering other forms of chronic illness.

The involvement of exercise and pets has proved beneficial in Alzheimer care in an innovative program at Parkside Manor nursing home in Wenatchee, Washington. But most Alzheimer patients are nursed at home in the United States and this can wreak havoc on a family. Utilizing a few shiatsu techniques—just on the feet or hands, perhaps—may offer a few reassuring moments in a day, and are worth a try.

The Swiss Red Cross asked me to give some shiatsu classes for visiting nurses caring for physically challenged senior citizens in their own homes. Physical benefits aside, shiatsu was appreciated for being a compassionate and noninvasive form of communication, and a special help for people who lived alone.

There's a lot more than just mechanics involved in shiatsu.

I've watched Berlin physiotherapist Inge Berlin perform miracles with a man in his seventies who'd had a stroke and was told by doctors he would never move again. Nonsense, said Inge. By combining physiotherapy techniques with deep breathing, shiatsu, visualization with ki energy, and a lot of humor, she had him out of bed in a matter of weeks, walking with the help of a cane and doing exercises on a mat on the floor.

In his excellent work *Ageless Body, Timeless Mind* physician-philosopher Deepak

Chopra, M.D., describes the 300 percent improvement in muscle strength, balance, and mental attitudes in senior citizens (aged eighty-seven to ninety-six) involved in weight training for eight weeks in experiments arranged by gerontologists from Tufts University in Boston.

In a later study the Tufts team showed how even the frailest of eighty- and ninety-year-olds swapped walkers for canes and walked or climbed stairs faster after only a few weeks of weight training for their legs (*New York Times*, June 23, 1994).

From these and other studies and observations, Dr. Chopra talks about the illusions of aging and the factors that retard aging, such as a daily routine, exercise, happiness, and a sound relationship.

But those are luxuries for many senior citizens whose lives are dogged by poverty, loneliness, and isolation from a society that no longer considers them of value.

I had my most intensive insight into the autumn of life while helping my mother recover from a heart attack and hip replacement surgery in Cape Town in 1992. Her physiotherapist and I alternated giving her isometric exercises until she could move from bed to wheelchair to walker to walking stick in four weeks. Coordinating breathing with movement proved very helpful, as she had a common tendency to hold her breath while exerting herself.

In her younger days, my mother was a great hockey and golf player and could dance the tango like a dream. I drew on all of this, utilizing familiar imagery and movements to help her walk. "Come on, Ma," I'd say. "You're on the dance floor. Now, then. Two steps forward, one back." Her spine would straighten, and a whole new energy would come through her. We laughed a lot.

My father underwent a series of surgeries before finally dying of leukemia, and he always loved me to give shiatsu to his shoulders, back, neck, hands, and feet, to ease pain and stiffness. He was also a terrific athlete in his youth—baseball, tennis, and then golf—and it was never hard to get him to talk about those days. His energy would surge under my fingertips when he reminisced.

In those moments when my mother felt frustrated about needing her children's help when she started to walk after her surgery, my brother Patrick and I would joke about life's pendulum and the bygone days when she taught us how to walk.

I gave biweekly classes to the medical staff at Avondrust retirement home for women, where my mother spent her final years in Cape Town. The response was deeply gratifying. Just by watching the interaction between the women and the nursing staff, I learned much more than I taught.

Negotiating stairs and corridors can be a major undertaking for the less agile, requiring skill and planning. Ability/disability is often related to the amount of time it takes to walk from point A to point B. A few moments of shiatsu can ease an aching joint or improve breathing, and can be done regularly by the attending nurses, by senior citizens themselves, or by a caring relative.

In all my classes we pinpointed typical, everyday needs and concentrated on a few key exercises. Not only did we work on one another, but, where possible, we involved some of the residents as models. Everyone found the exercises easy to learn, easy to apply. Some of the nurses found time to give ten-minute sessions every day or so.

Everyone commented on the side benefits of comfortable, pain-free touching, and in utilizing some of the principles of shiatsu to help with tasks like lifting the chronically ill in and out of bed or into a wheelchair, or helping someone wash, bathe, or dress.

This experience reinforced my belief that health care givers do wonders for themselves and their patients if they can utilize exercises that give joy as well as relief, to offset many of the painful or uncomfortable tasks often associated with hospital or nursing home care. This is a general rule but is even more important in chronic care.

The very frail need only a minimum of pressure. Work very gently. Variations on the following basic techniques will come with practice, depending, of course, on the person's degree of flexibility and health. With the very thin or chronically bedridden, the application of soft, sweet-smelling lotions on hands, feet, back, and buttocks may be more comfortable and comforting than shiatsu.

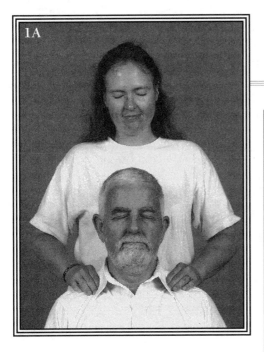

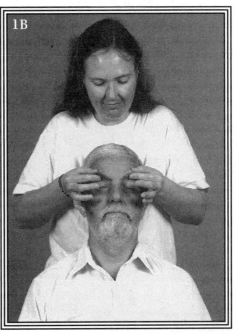

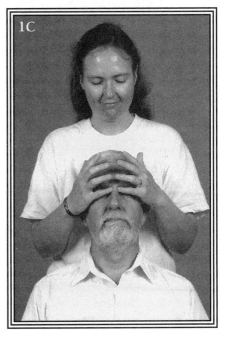

General Techniques for Common Pains or Prevention, or for the Chronically Ill or Physically Challenged of Any Age

1. *Head and Shoulders* (when person is seated or in a wheelchair).

1A. Squeeze shoulders gently, release gently.

1B. Squeeze eyebrows.

1C. Pinch bridge of nose. Press and release.

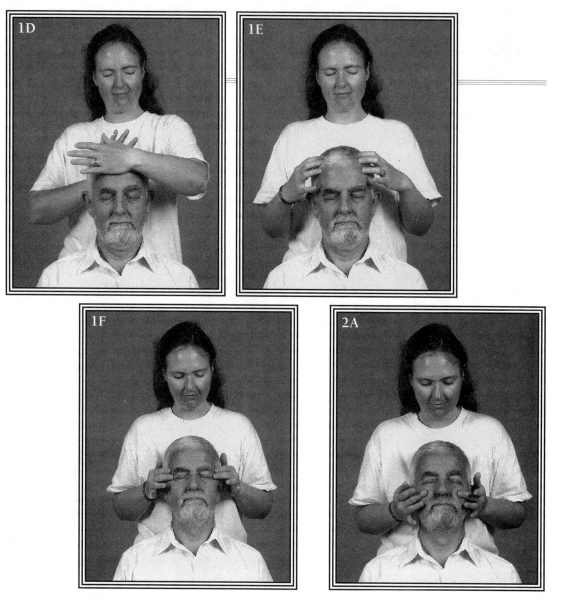

1D. Press and release head, slowly and gently.

1E. Press fingertips over head to neck (see headaches, p. 23).

1F. Draw slow, gentle circles at temples.
Benefits headaches, tight neck and shoulders, and eyestrain.

2. *Face:*

2A. Apply pressure under cheekbones.

2B. Apply pressure on either side of nostrils (see p. 32).
Benefits congestions from sinus, colds, and poor breathing.

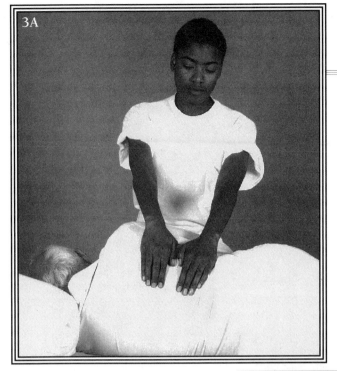

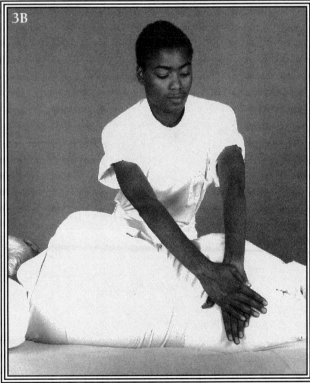

3. *Back* (in side position):

3A. Work down either side of spine using firm finger pressure and lean back slightly, keeping your arms straight.

3B. Press hands against sacrum. *Benefits back pain, constipation, insomnia.*

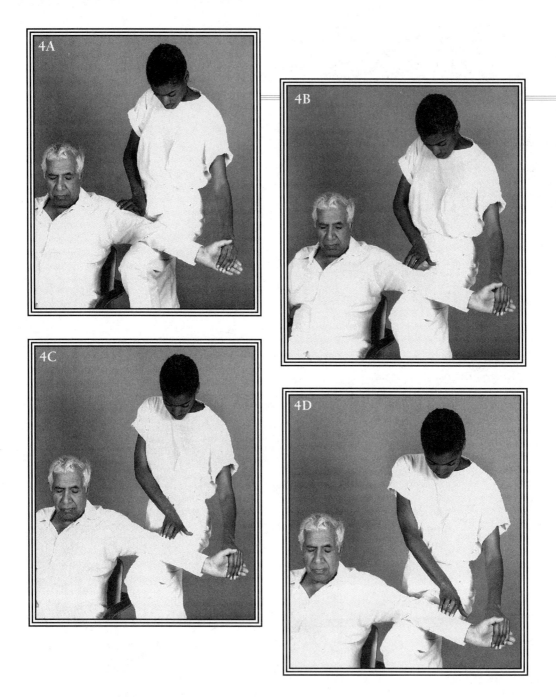

4. *Arms:*

4A–D. Stretch arm and support palm up. Hold patient's thumb open and press line from shoulder to thumb (see pp. 29–31).

Benefits breathing problems—chronic asthma, allergies, fluid on the lungs.

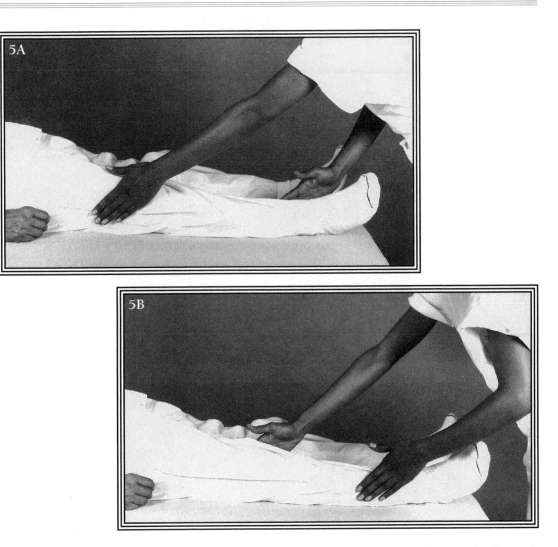

5. *Feet, Legs, and Hands:* Follow sequence for feet and hands (pp. 101–104).
Stroke up legs in alternate directions (up on inside, down on outside).
Benefits circulation, tired legs, stiff hands. Can be done on arthritic patients, but work gently.

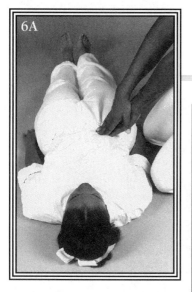

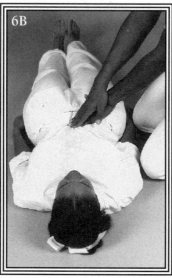

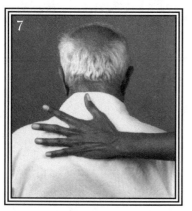

6A–C. *Abdominal work:* Work up the ascending colon, across the transverse, and down the descending colon. Brisk rolling of fingers in wave-like motion for constipation. Slower movement for diarrhea.

Benefits constipation, diarrhea, gas, abdominal discomfort (see Constipation, p. 34).

7. *Additional techniques for stress or sadness:* Visualize a circle encompassing the top three thoracic vertebrae. Press gently with your thumbs, or press and support with the palm of your hand.

Benefits tight breathing due to sadness or stress.

Practice these techniques gently and evenly. You'll soon discover which techniques feel most comfortable and helpful for you and your loved ones, friends, or patients. Sometimes it takes only five minutes to give compassionate shiatsu and ease pain or discomfort.

F. WORKING WITH THE DYING

I spent some days at the bedside of a dying friend who received shiatsu from me during the final months of her terminal breast and lung cancer. She was a confrontational sort of person, a journalist and activist, a street fighter in many ways. She knew she was going to die and it frustrated her. She scorned religious beliefs and felt all she wanted to do was take her backpack and go off hiking in the New England fall and die amidst the trees with their glorious colors. She was too sick to leave her bed so we talked about her next "journey."

"Don't feel this is the end," I said. "Death is like swapping one setting for another. And they probably have some challenge lined up for you on the other side, my friend. You'll go on learning and developing. You're too bloody-minded to evaporate or go floating off on a cloud!"

"I like that," she laughed.

She died a month later.

I repeated this story in one of my classes, and a voice piped up, "What use was shiatsu? Your friend died."

"Ah, but shiatsu combined with our wonderful discussions brought an inner healing and reconciliation," I said, adding, "and the experience enriched me."

There's an art in helping people die. Nurses, in particular, have taught me a lot about the practical side of being there, of directness, and of tuning in logically to the belief system of the dying person.

There's a marvelous nun called Sister Loretta Palamara who wanders around the hospice at Cabrini Hospital in New York City at night, dressed as a clown or Charlie Chaplin.

She and others who help ease the passage of the dying with a mixture of humor, compassion, and a ready ear often underline the ability of an outsider to deal with death more easily than the families of the dying can. Barriers sometimes drop. There's no past baggage to deal with. Priorities swing into focus.

People who work with the dying all stress the importance of a compassionate touch, especially when words are no longer appropriate. Recently, Sister Loretta sat in her clown outfit, using mime instead of words, beside a dying man who had experienced weeks of pain. After fifteen minutes he told her the pain had gone.

Even if you have practiced little in this book except the techniques for feet and hands, you can do a lot to help ease pain, and comfort a dying relative or friend, young or old.

Depending on the nature of the illness or recent surgery, just follow the simple shiatsu routines outlined in earlier sections. Or you can rub soft cream on their hands, feet, or back—especially if they are stiff and uncomfortable from lying in bed for long periods. You won't do any harm, and you can continue doing this even if your loved ones are in a coma or unconscious. We're told the sense of hearing is the last sense to go, so play their favorite music to them, through a Walkman if necessary.

There's nothing more distressing than to peep through the half-open door of a hospital room and see members of a family standing awkwardly around the bed of a dying relative, whispering, shuffling, averting their eyes, or staring blankly at the dying person or the machines beside the bed.

And then there's a general noisy exodus as everyone clatters out of the room when visiting time is up, and the person dies an hour later when no one is around.

In our so-called civilized Western cultures, except for those still linked to traditional customs and practices, we're clumsy around death. In the United States funeral homes charge a fortune to embalm and euphemize death in ways that are not practiced elsewhere in the world.

We've lost many of the rituals of our ancestors, rituals that help the soul to journey on and the bereaved to cope with the process of mourning. The Jewish practice of sitting shivah for seven days after a person dies provides a practical framework or structure for grief and mourning. The New Orleans jazz funeral has its origin in many of the rituals of Africa, where burials are seen as collective efforts and onlookers join in the funeral procession as it passes by, whether they knew the deceased or not. Growing up in South Africa, I learned about ancestor worship, or the recognition of a "living dead." I was moved by one particular funeral where chief mourners used the coffin like a table for their prayer books, and slapped it with their hands while addressing the departed directly by name in eulogies, a vigorous departure from our polite Anglo funerals where people keep their distance from the coffin. The haunting Xhosa burial chant "Hamba Kahle"—"Go Well"—is also a form of adieu for a living friend.

Eastern religions have intricate rituals surrounding death and dying, as do many indigenous peoples.

But more and more people are creating their own rituals, especially for loved ones dying young from AIDS or cancer. Friends and family members gather to quote poems and share memories, scatter ashes, plant trees or rose gardens, or create scholarships or grants to fund a continuation of the work or cause of the loved one. Creating a sense of continuity seems to be a key here to overcome a feeling of desolation, desertion, abandonment, unresolve, grief, and loss.

A fascinating Mexican and Mexican-American custom is *El Día de los Muertos* (Day of the Dead) each November 1 and 2 (All Saints' and All Souls' Days). The practice is rooted in Aztec rituals, with parallels in other rituals celebrating the dead, like the ancient Celtic Halloween on October 31.

On *Día de los Muertos* families collect in cemeteries to clean and adorn graves with flowers and to picnic around the grave. Catholic Europe practices variations of this custom, depending on location, like *Allerheiligen* in parts of Germany and Switzerland, when families place flowers on graves after Mass.

Cultures share similar baking customs, like the Mexican *pan de muertos* and the German *Seelenbrot*.

As my family straddles three continents (the U.S., Britain, South Africa), deaths have been scattered affairs, involving long-distance phone calls and last-minute long-distance travel, and with no sense of family continuity in any one place.

I discussed death openly with both my parents. I knew about their funeral wishes and that helped a lot.

My parents died exactly five weeks apart at the end of 1993. My father died in Florida U.S.A., and my mother in Cape Town, South Africa. They had been divorced for almost forty years.

Rose petals provided an important link in their funeral rituals. I scattered rose petals over my father's ashes in the Gulf of Mexico and brought petals from those same roses home with me to Texas. Little did I know I'd be taking some of them to Cape Town a month later to bury with my mother, along with roses from the garden of the Dominican convent with which she was associated, and petals from my cousin Geoff's garden in Winchester, England. I saved some of the collection to bring home and later to scatter on the grave where her grandparents and brother are buried in their beloved Cornwall.

My Aunt Patty tossed a shot of bourbon into the waves after my brother Jimmy and I scattered my father's ashes: he loved his sundowner. I buried an Earl Grey tea bag with my mother, an inveterate tea drinker. I was inspired by the Zen Buddhist ritual of placing a bowl of rice and chopsticks near the ashes of the departed, to feed the soul as it travels on.

It was my way of saying farewell.

BIBLIOGRAPHY
AND
SUGGESTED READING

Shiatsu

Masunaga, Shizuto with Wataru Ohashi. *Zen Shiatsu: How to Harmonize Yin and Yang for Better Health.* Tokyo: Japan Publications, 1977 (distributed by Harper & Row USA).

Ohashi, Wataru. *Do-It-Yourself Shiatsu: How to Perform the Ancient Japanese Art of "Acupuncture Without Needles."* New York: EP Dutton, 1976.

Chinese Medicine

Kaptchuk, Ted J. *The Web That Has No Weaver: Understanding Chinese Medicine.* New York: Congdon & Weed, Inc., 1983.

Hatha Yoga

White, Ganga with Anna Forrest. *Double Yoga: A New System for Total Body Health.* New York: Penguin Books, 1981.

Eastern and Western Medicine

Chopra, Deepak. *Ageless Body, Timeless Mind: The Quantum Alternative to Growing Old.* New York: Crown Publishers, 1993.

Cousins, Norman. *Anatomy of an Illness.* New York: Bantam Books, 1983.

Eisenberg, David and Thomas L. Wright. *Encounters with Qi.* New York: Penguin Books, 1987.

Mann, Felix. *Atlas of Acupuncture: Points and Meridians in a Relation to Surface Anatomy.* London: William Heinemann Medical Books, 1990.

Monte, Tom and the editors of EastWest Natural Health. *World Medicine: The East-West Guide to Healing Your Body.* New York: Tarcher/Perigee Books, 1993.

Rosenbaum, E. *The Doctor.* New York: Ivy Books, 1988.

Stanway, Andrew. *Alternative Medicine: A Guide to Natural Therapies.* London: Bloomsbury Books, 1980.

The Visual Encyclopedia of Natural Healing—A Step-by-Step Pictorial Guide to Solving 100 Everyday Health Problems. Emmaus, PA: Rodale Press, Inc., 1991.

Women and Medicine:

Andrews, Lynn V. *Medicine Woman.* San Francisco: Harper & Row, 1981.

Greer, Germaine. *The Change: Women, Aging, and the Menopause.* New York: Fawcett Columbine, 1991.

Lark, Susan M. *The Menopause Self-Help Book.* Berkeley, CA: Celestial Arts, 1990.

Love, Susan M. and Karen Lindsey. *Dr. Susan Love's Breast Book.* Reading, MA: Addison-Wesley, 1991.

Sheehy, Gail. *The Silent Passage.* New York: Pocket Books, 1993.

Mythology

West, John O. *Mexican-American Folklore.* Little Rock, AK: August House, 1988.

INDEX

═══════

About the Author

Pamela Ferguson is a shiatsu instructor, registered massage therapist, and author of half a dozen books published in the US, UK, and Canada during her years in journalism. Born in Chihuahua, Mexico, and raised in Cape Town, South Africa, she received her shiatsu training from Pauline Sasaki, Esther Turnbull, and Ohashi at the Shiatsu Education Center in New York, where she has also taught. She also attended the Asten Center of Natural Therapeutics in Dallas, Texas. She pioneered shiatsu teaching in five hospitals, including the Psychiatrische Klinik Sanatorium Kilchberg near Zurich, and the School of Physiotherapy at Bern's Inselspital, and St. Vincent's in New York. She teaches annually at Berlin's Zentrum fur Chinesische Medizin, Schule fur Shiatsu Berlin Hamburg, Shiatsu-Zentrum Edith Storch, and at schools in Dresden and Winterthur.

She is a member of the African National Congress and President of the Breast Cancer Action Group (of the US) and combines health and political activism in her travels.

About the Photographer

Alison Russell is a Dallas, Texas, photographer.